Lung Cancer Screening

Janelle V. Baptiste • Richard M. Schwartzstein
Carey C. Thomson

Editors

Lung Cancer Screening

Practical Aspects for Primary Care

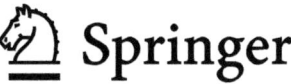 Springer

Editors
Janelle V. Baptiste
Division of Pulmonary
Critical Care & Sleep Medicine
Beth Israel Deaconess Medical Center
Harvard Medical School
Boston, MA, USA

Richard M. Schwartzstein
Division of Pulmonary
Critical Care and Sleep Medicine
Beth Israel Deaconess Medical Center
Harvard Medical School
Boston, MA, USA

Carey C. Thomson
Division of Pulmonary and Critical Care
Medicine
Mt Auburn Hospital/Beth Israel
Lahey Health
Harvard Medical School
Boston, MA, USA

ISBN 978-3-031-10661-3   ISBN 978-3-031-10662-0   (eBook)
https://doi.org/10.1007/978-3-031-10662-0

This Springer imprint is published by the registered company Springer Nature Switzerland AG
The registered company address is: Gewerbestrasse 11, 6330 Cham, Switzerland

Introduction

The role of primary care practitioners (PCP) in encouraging high-risk individuals to consider participating in screening is central to any screening program [1]. Primary care recommendations have a significant influence on screening participation [2, 3]. Primary care providers are often the first point of contact for a patient and provide most preventive health care to patients. The essential role of PCPs in patient engagement with lung cancer screening (LCS) is demonstrated in a retrospective cohort analysis which showed that patient uptake was more likely if the patient had seen his or her own general practitioner than if they had not (8.5% versus 4.7%, $p < 0.0001$) [4]. Involvement of PCPs in LCS can enhance both the ease of identifying and recruiting eligible individuals for LCS and provide the financial resources necessary to implement, perform, and sustain LCS. However, PCPs face significant barriers in performing LCS. In the cross-sectional survey by Spalluto et al. of providers, staff, and administrators in radiology and primary care at a single Veterans Affairs Medical Center, radiology health professions had higher levels of readiness for change for implementation of LCS than those in primary care [5]. These results were likely due to more organizational barriers perceived in primary care in implementing LCS. Acknowledging the barriers to implementing and sustaining LCS programs in primary care; clinical and research experts in Pulmonary medicine, Chest radiology, Primary care medicine, and LCS program implementation have collaborated in the writing of this book, *Lung Cancer Screening: Practical Aspects for Primary Care*.

Lung cancer remains the deadliest cancer worldwide for male and female individuals combined. In Chap. 1, Baldwin and colleagues will take us through the epidemiology of lung cancer worldwide. However, in the United States alone, almost one quarter of all estimated deaths from cancer in 2021 were estimated to be due to lung cancer [6]. Lung cancer is predicted to remain the leading cause of US cancer-related deaths well into 2040 [7]. Neither of these projections, however, take into account the impact of the ongoing coronavirus disease 2019 (COVID-19) pandemic on cancer-related deaths. It is expected that deaths from cancer will ultimately increase as a result of delays in diagnosis and treatment caused by the shutdowns during the COVID-19 pandemic.

Despite this sobering estimate, lung cancer deaths are on a continuous decline. The annual rate at which lung cancer deaths are falling has accelerated in recent years from 3.1% to 5.5% in men and from 1.8% to 4.4% in women, during the period of 2009 to 2018 [6]. The decline in lung cancer deaths is largely due to reductions in tobacco cigarette smoking and improvements in the treatment of lung cancer.

The decline in tobacco cigarette smoking is thought to be from improved tobacco control efforts in the United States following from the landmark 1964, First Surgeon General's Report, on the serious health consequences of smoking [8, 9]. Tobacco smoking still remains the number one cause for lung cancer deaths. In the United States alone, 34 million adults were estimated to still smoke in 2019; and while this represents a continued decline in the numbers of current smokers it continues to place a large fraction of the population at risk for lung cancer [10].

In regions of the world with fewer resources, pollutants related to fuel used for cooking are playing an increasing role in the global burden of lung cancer. In the United States, non-smoking-related lung cancer deaths have now surpassed lung cancer deaths from second-hand smoking and with women having a larger fraction of non-smoking-related lung cancer than men [7, 11].

There is also a growing disparity in smoking trends in the United States. Many vulnerable populations have not experienced similar declines in prevalence of cigarette smoking, and a larger fraction of these groups remain at high risk [12]. Disparities in health which can occur in relation to race and ethnicity, sex, gender and gender identity, mental health, disability, socioeconomic status, and geographical location can occur in lung cancer diagnosis, treatment, and mortality outcomes and potentially exacerbate disparities in LCS [13]. In Chap. 2, Steiling and coauthor provide us with a comprehensive review of health disparities in LCS and the factors associated with lower rates of LCS.

Although primary prevention of lung cancer through smoking cessation is key to reducing mortality from lung cancer, deaths from lung cancer in former smokers do not demonstrate the same benefit as primary prevention. Lung cancer survival is also closely related to the stage at diagnosis, that is, its prognosis is more favorable when diagnosed at an earlier stage [14]. Secondary prevention, therefore, is also needed to decrease cancer-specific deaths. Secondary prevention by screening for lung cancer with low-dose chest tomography (LDCT) is shown to reduce cancer-specific deaths in current and former tobacco cigarette smokers with the detection of early-stage lung cancer. Thomson et al. review the evidence base for LCS in Chap. 3, including a review of the United States National Lung Screening Trial (NLST) and the Dutch-Belgium Randomized Lung Cancer Screening Trial (Nederlands-Leuvens Longkanker Screenings Onderzoek, NELSON), both having shown a reduction in lung cancer-specific mortality with the use of LDCT [1]. In the

NLST, 20% fewer people in the LDCT screening arm died of lung cancer than the chest radiograph arm, and overall mortality was reduced by 7% [15–17]. The NELSON trial, published 10 years later, showed that 26% fewer males died from lung cancer by screening with LDCT.

The results from the NLST very quickly led to several US advisory organizations, including the US Preventive Services Task Force (USPSTF), and National Comprehensive Cancer Network (NCCN), recommending LCS [18, 19]. Implementation of LCS programs across the United States followed from these recommendations. Early 2015, the Affordable Care Act mandated that private insurance companies must cover screening with LDCT for eligible populations in keeping with the USPSTF guideline; Centers for Medicare and Medicaid Services (CMS) followed later that year with approval for payment coverage for LCS for high-risk Medicare beneficiaries [20]. Both payer systems require tobacco cessation and shared decision-making documentation for payment. The economics around LCS in the United States is complex and mandates knowledge and understanding of LCS coverage policies and eligibility criteria, billing, and reimbursement of follow-up testing. Acknowledging these complexities, Michaud and coauthor provide PCPs with a reference guide on LCS economics and billing in Chap. 4.

The impact of LCS outside of these two large randomized trials, however, has not carried over into the real-world setting. The impact of real-world LCS programs on population-based mortality trends remains small [21]. This is mainly due to the low uptake of LDCT screening by the target population and the challenges with implementing LCS into healthcare settings. Only a small percentage of the eligible US population report having received LDCT screening. Literature assessing the readiness of primary care clinics to implement LDCT programs found that only 10% of respondents had LCS available in their practice [22]. Implementation challenges affect LCS in clinical practice. The barriers to implementation of LCS in clinical practice arise at multiple levels of healthcare delivery. Research looking at the barriers and facilitators to implementing evidence-based interventions into real-world settings and the influence on outcomes shows that many interventions found to be effective in research often fail to translate into meaningful patient care outcomes in real-world settings [23].

Primary care is recognized as both paramount and challenged in identifying individuals for LCS. Many factors need to be considered when implementing LCS in primary care and Baptiste et al. identify some of the facilitators and challenges to implementation in Chap. 4. Implementing LCS in primary care is a process which begins with correctly identifying and determining an individual's eligibility for screening. Barta and coauthor propose leveraging the electronic health record (EHR) to facilitate LCS in primary care-driven programs while also providing critical support to centralized programs through improvement of EHR documentation. CMS coverage of LCS also has several requirements which creates specific challenges for PCP. Roelke and coauthors, in their chapter, explore the necessary components of the shared decision-making discussion, tobacco cessation counseling, and benefits and harms within the context of LCS.

Radiologists have been involved in LCS for many years and have a lot of experience from years of developing breast cancer screening programs. An effective high-quality LCS program requires multidisciplinary teams with broad expertise. Dyer and coauthor, from the department of radiology, provide a practical approach in Chap. 6 to ordering, interpreting, reporting, and tracking results of LCS and review the guidelines for managing incidental findings.

Lung Cancer Screening: Practical Aspects for Primary Care recognizes the challenges faced by those in primary care in establishing LCS and the need for more practical guidance from experts in the field of LCS. A broad range of views and ideas are presented on LCS. This book is written for primary care, which is inclusive of physicians, advanced practice providers, nurses, staff, administrators, and leadership. We hope that this book will provide a roadmap to the creation of a successful LCS program that has the potential to save countless lives.

References

1. Rankin NM, McWilliams A, Marshall HM. Lung cancer screening implementation: complexities and priorities. Respirology. 2020;25 Suppl 2:5–23.
2. Draucker CB, Rawl SM, Vode E, Carter-Harris L. Understanding the decision to screen for lung cancer or not: a qualitative analysis. Health Expect. 2019;22(6):1314–21.
3. Carter-Harris L, Slaven JE Jr, Monahan PO, Shedd-Steele R, Hanna N, Rawl SM. Understanding lung cancer screening behavior: racial, gender, and geographic differences among Indiana long-term smokers. Prev Med Rep. 2018;10:49–54.
4. Li J, Chung S, Wei EK, Luft HS. New recommendation and coverage of low-dose computed tomography for lung cancer screening: uptake has increased but is still low. BMC Health Serv Res. 2018;18(1):525.
5. Spalluto LB, Lewis JA, Stolldorf D, Yeh VM, Callaway-Lane C, Wiener RS, Slatore CG, Yankelevitz DF, Henschke CI, Vogus TJ, Massion PP, Moghanaki D, Roumie CL. Organizational readiness for lung cancer screening: a cross-sectional evaluation at a Veterans Affairs Medical Center. J Am Coll Radiol. 2021;18(6):809–19. https://doi.org/10.1016/j.jacr.2020.12.010. Epub 2021 Jan 7. Erratum in: J Am Coll Radiol. 2021;18(9):1371. PMID: 33421372; PMCID: PMC8180484.
6. Siegel RL, Miller KD, Fuchs HE, Jemal A. Cancer statistics, 2021. CA Cancer J Clin. 2021;71(1):7–33. https://doi.org/10.3322/caac.21654. Epub 2021 Jan 12. Erratum in: CA Cancer J Clin. 2021;71(4):359.
7. Rahib L, Wehner MR, Matrisian LM, Nead KT. Estimated projection of US cancer incidence and death to 2040. JAMA Netw Open. 2021;4(4):e214708.
8. Holford TR, Meza R, Warner KE, Meernik C, Jeon J, Moolgavkar SH, Levy DT. Tobacco control and the reduction in smoking-related premature deaths in the United States, 1964-2012. JAMA. 2014;311(2):164–71.

9. Warner KE, Sexton DW, Gillespie BW, Levy DT, Chaloupka FJ. Impact of tobacco control on adult per capita cigarette consumption in the United States. Am J Public Health. 2014;104(1):83–9.

10. Cornelius ME, Wang TW, Jamal A, Loretan C, Neff L. Tobacco product use among adults—United States, 2019. Morb Mort Wkly Rep. 2020;69(46):1736–42.

11. Islami F, Goding Sauer A, Miller KD, et al. Proportion and number of cancer cases and deaths attributable to potentially modifiable factors in the United States in 2014. CA Cancer J Clin. 2018;68:31–54.

12. Doogan NJ, Roberts ME, Wewers ME, Stanton CA, Keith DR, Gaalema DE, Kurti AN, Redner R, Cepeda-Benito A, Bunn JY, Lopez AA, Higgins ST. A growing geographic disparity: rural and urban cigarette smoking trends in the United States. Prev Med. 2017;104:79–85.

13. HHS action plan to reduce racial and ethnic health disparities. https://www.minorityhealth.hhs.gov/assets/pdf/hhs/HHS_Plan_complete.pdf.

14. Zhou Q, Fan Y, Wu N, Huang Y, Wang Y, Li L, Liu J, Wang X, Li W, Qiao Y. Demonstration program of population-based lung cancer screening in China: rationale and study design. Thorac Cancer. 2014;5(3):197–203.

15. Aberle DR, Adams AM, Berg CD, et al. National Lung Screening Trial Research Team. Reduced lung-cancer mortality with low-dose computed tomographic screening. N Engl J Med. 2011;365(5):395–409.

16. Church TR, Black WC, Aberle DR, et al. National Lung Screening Trial Research Team. Results of initial low-dose computed tomographic screening for lung cancer. N Engl J Med. 2013;368(21):1980–91.

17. Aberle DR, DeMello S, Berg CD, et al. National Lung Screening Trial Research Team. Results of the two incidence screenings in the National Lung Screening Trial. N Engl J Med. 2013;369(10):920–31.

18. Clinical summary: lung cancer: screening. U.S. Preventive Services Task Force. 2014. https://www.uspreventiveservicestaskforce.org/Page/Document/ClinicalSummaryFinal/lung-cancer-screening.

19. Wood DE, Kazerooni EA, Baum SL, Eapen GA, Ettinger DS, Hou L, Jackman DM, Klippenstein D, Kumar R, Lackner RP, Leard LE, Lennes IT, Leung ANC, Makani SS, Massion PP, Mazzone P, Merritt RE, Meyers BF, Midthun DE, Pipavath S, Pratt C, Reddy C, Reid ME, Rotter AJ, Sachs PB, Schabath MB, Schiebler ML, Tong BC, Travis WD, Wei B, Yang SC, Gregory KM, Hughes M. Lung Cancer Screening, Version 3. NCCN clinical practice guidelines in oncology. J Natl Compr Cancer Netw. 2018;16(4):412–41.

20. Bindman A. JAMA forum: lung cancer screening and evidence-based policy. JAMA. 2015;313(1):17–8.

21. Howlader N, Forjaz G, Mooradian MJ, Meza R, Kong CY, Cronin KA, Mariotto AB, Lowy DR, Feuer EJ. The effect of advances in lung-cancer treatment on population mortality. N Engl J Med. 2020;383(7):640–9.

22. Volk RJ, Foxhall LE. Readiness of primary care clinicians to implement lung cancer screening programs. Prev Med Rep. 2015;2:717–9.

23. Liang S, Kegler MC, Cotter M, Emily P, Beasley D, Hermstad A, Morton R, Martinez J, Riehman K. Integrating evidence-based practices for increasing cancer screenings in safety net health systems: a multiple case study using the Consolidated Framework for Implementation Research. Implement Sci. 2016;11:109. https://doi.org/10.1186/s13012-016-0477-4. Erratum in: Implement Sci. 2016;11(1):130. PMID: 27485452; PMCID: PMC4970264.

Division of Pulmonary   Janelle V. Baptiste
Critical Care and Sleep Medicine
Beth Israel Deaconess Medical Center
Harvard Medical School
Boston, MA, USA

Division of Pulmonary   Richard M. Schwartzstein
Critical Care and Sleep Medicine
Beth Israel Deaconess Medical Center
Harvard Medical School
Boston, MA, USA

Division of Pulmonary and Critical Care Medicine   Carey C. Thomson
Mt Auburn Hospital/Beth Israel Lahey Health
Harvard Medical School
Boston, MA, USA

Contents

Chapter 1
Epidemiology of Lung Cancer and Risk Factors

Amna Burzić, Helen Morgan, and David Baldwin

1.1 Epidemiology of Lung Cancer

Worldwide, lung cancer is the second most common cancer diagnosis, only behind female breast cancer, and is the leading cause of cancer-related death. The World Health Organization (WHO) estimated 2.21 million cases of lung cancer and 1.8 million lung cancer-related deaths in 2020 [1]. Although there has been a decline in overall incidence worldwide, lung cancer rates show significant geographic diversity and gender disparities. As nearly 80% of lung cancer is attributable to cigarette smoking [2], the observed trends primarily reflect the maturity of the tobacco epidemic worldwide [3].

1.1.1 Incidence

Lung cancer made up an estimated 11.4% of total cancer cases for both sexes worldwide in 2020. There is significant geographical variation worldwide in lung cancer incidence rates, as shown in Fig. 1.1. More developed countries tend to have a

A. Burzić
Department of Respiratory Medicine, David Evans Centre, City Hospital Campus, Nottingham University Hospitals NHS Trust, Nottingham, England

H. Morgan (✉) · D. Baldwin
Department of Respiratory Medicine, David Evans Centre, City Hospital Campus, Nottingham University Hospitals NHS Trust, Nottingham, England

Division of Epidemiology and Public Health, University of Nottingham, Nottingham, England
e-mail: helen.morgan@nottingham.ac.uk

© The Author(s), under exclusive license to Springer Nature Switzerland AG 2022
J. V. Baptiste et al. (eds.), *Lung Cancer Screening*, https://doi.org/10.1007/978-3-031-10662-0_1

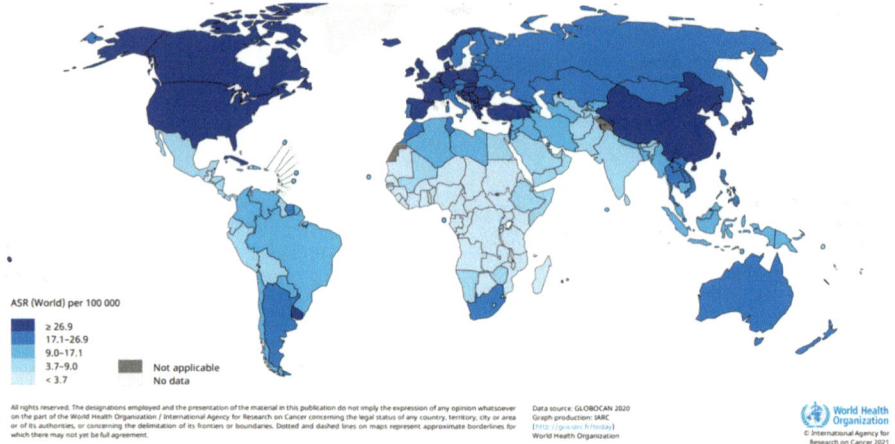

Fig. 1.1 Estimated age-standardised incidence rates for lung cancer in 2020, both sexes. (With permissions from Cancer Today, International Agency for Research on Cancer [1])

higher incidence compared with less developed countries (39.0 vs. 10.3 per 100,000 in males; 18.2 vs. 4.2 per 100,000 in females). Polynesia had the highest observed incidence rate worldwide, 37.3 per 100,000. North America and Europe account for a third of lung cancer worldwide [4].

Given the lead time between onset of smoking and development of lung cancer, incidence and prevalence rates often reflect changes in smoking patterns decades earlier. In the United Kingdom (UK) overall incidence has been decreasing since the 1970s, however in recent years this has started to plateau, with a 1% increase over the last decade. For males, rates have continued to decrease by around a third in this time. In females however, the incidence continues to increase by nearly the same amount, with a third more cases annually in 2017 compared with 1993 [5] (Fig. 1.2). Similarly, in mainland Europe, incidence in men has been decreasing since the early 1990s but rates continue to increase in women. Owing to the earlier stage of smoking trends in Eastern Europe, rates continue to increase [6]. In the USA, lung cancer incidence in males peaked in the 1980s, with a slow decline since (Fig. 1.3). For females, the same trends were observed around 20 years later [7].

1.1.2 Mortality

In 2020, lung cancer is estimated to have caused 1.79 million deaths (18.0% of total cancer deaths) worldwide [4]. Mortality rates closely follow incidence, and we see a similar worldwide variation with greater mortality in more developed countries than less developed. Age-standardised mortality rates in more developed countries are nearly double that of the least developed (31.6 vs. 13.7 per 100,000 in males) [4]. Following the pattern of cigarette smoking and incidence, male lung cancer

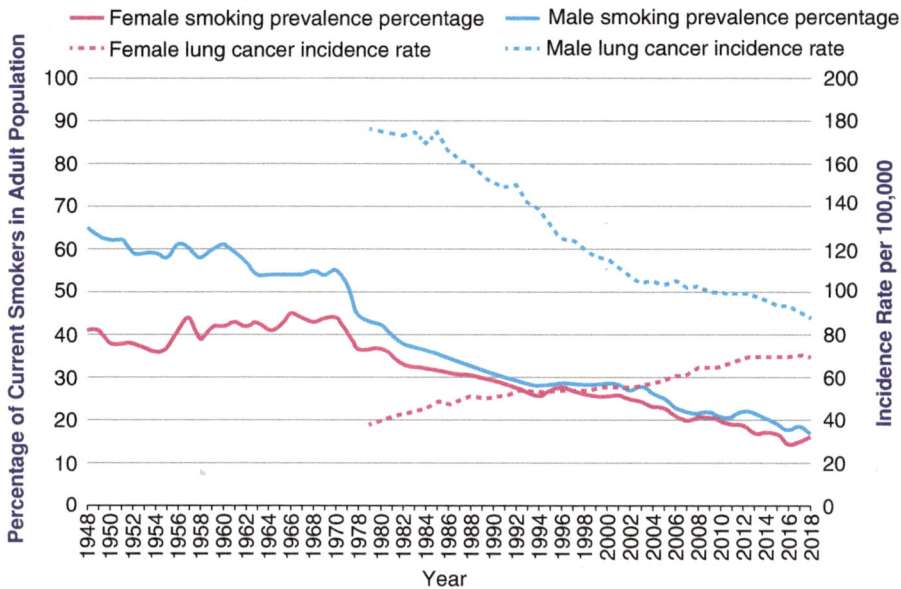

Fig. 1.2 Smoking prevalence and age-standardised incidence rates for lung cancer in Great Britain, 1948–2018. (With permissions from Cancer Research UK [5])

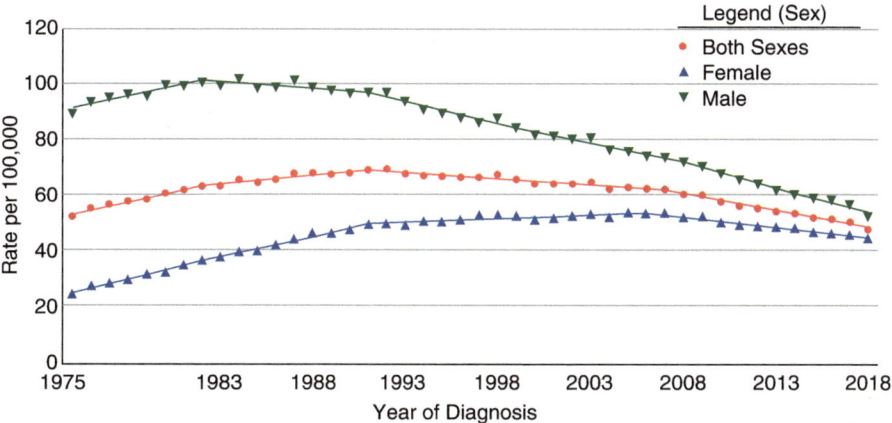

Fig. 1.3 SEER (Surveillance, Epidemiology and End Results) age-adjusted lung cancer incidence rate per 100,000 in the United States 1975–2018. (With permissions from SEER Explorer [7])

mortality has been steadily declining since 2000, whereas it has been increasing in women. The USA, where mortality has also been decreasing in women, is an exception in this regard [8].

Survival in lung cancer is closely related to stage of disease at presentation. Worldwide, age-standardised 5-year survival in 2014 ranged from less than 10%

(Thailand, Brazil, Bulgaria and India) to 32.9% (Japan). Most countries fall between 10% and 20%. In the USA, 5-year survival was 21.2%, and 13.3% in the UK [9]. There have been gains in survival since 1995, although these data also show wide geographic variability. In the USA, Canada and several European countries including the UK, survival has increased by 5–10% [10]. Survival in China and Korea increased by more than 10% during this time [9].

1.1.3   Stage at Presentation

Unfortunately, most people present for care when lung cancer is at an advanced stage, when treatment intent is one of disease control rather than cure. In the USA, 21.5% of people present with localised disease, 21.4% with regional, and 50.7% with distant metastatic disease [7]. This is similar to data from the UK, with 28.9% at stages I and II, 21.6% at stage III, and 49.5% at stage IV. Survival is closely linked to stage at diagnosis; in England 5-year survival was 58.7%, 35.3%, 13.6% and 3.4% for stages I–IV, respectively [11]. In the USA, 5-year survival was 57.2% for localised disease, 29.7% for regional and 5.1% for distant disease [7].

1.1.4   Histological Subtypes

Lung cancer is divided into two main histological subtypes: non-small cell lung cancer (NSCLC), which makes up around 85% of tumours, and small cell lung cancer (SCLC), which accounts for roughly 15%. NSCLC is further divided into adenocarcinoma, squamous cell carcinoma and large cell carcinoma [12]. Historically, squamous cell carcinoma was the most common histological subtype, but since the 1990s the incidence of adenocarcinoma has been increasing, and it is now the most common type in North America, Europe and Japan. These changes are thought to be due to changes in the type of cigarettes smoked (e.g. filtered, low tar) as well as genetic predisposition [6, 13].

1.2   Lung Cancer Risk Factors

1.2.1   Demographic Factors

Although global lung cancer incidence and mortality rates in males are approximately double those in females, the relative rates are mostly a reflection of historical smoking rates in men and women. Some evidence suggests that women may be more susceptible to lung cancer [14]. Rates are higher in non-smoking females than males, and there is evidence that women with a 40 pack-year smoking history are three times more likely to develop lung cancer than males with the same smoking history [15]. As described previously, incidence has been increasing in women while decreasing in men. Generally, women began smoking later in the twentieth century than men, and cessation in smoking also lagged behind that seen in men. This is likely responsible for the later peak in lung cancer incidence (Fig. 1.2).

Increasing age is strongly also associated with increased incidence. The median age at presentation with lung cancer is 70 for both men and women [14]. The age adjusted rates for lung cancer increases from 44.3 per 100,000 in age 40–64, to 258.2 in 65–74, and 368.1 in age 75 and over [7].

1.2.2 Smoking

The link between lung cancer and smoking is well established, with the first evidence being published in the 1950s [16]. In Europe, an estimated 87% of lung cancers in males versus 70% in females are caused by cigarette smoking [17]. The differing trends in smoking worldwide also at least partially explain the variation in lung cancer rates between countries [4]. In the west, smoking rates in men have declined since the 1950s (Fig. 1.2). After a lag, we observe a drop in lung cancer incidence since the 1970s. As the peak in smoking occurred later in women, so did the peak in incidence, with some countries only recently observing a decline in female incidence [2].

Socioeconomic status (SES) also significantly contributes to variation in smoking rates within countries. People of lower SES are more likely to smoke. In the USA, people living in poverty smoke for nearly twice as many years as people with a high income [18]. In the UK, 27% of those in the lowest SES category smoke, compared with 8% in the highest SES group [19]. This correlates with higher rates of lung cancer in those with the fewest financial resources. Rates are 174% higher for women in the lowest socioeconomic group compared with the highest, with similar variation seen for men (168% higher rates for men with the fewest financial resources) [5].

Smoking cessation substantially reduces the risk of death from lung cancer, with greater effects being seen in those who stop at a younger age. For those who stop smoking before middle age, the risk of lung cancer falls by more than 90% [2]. Studies have shown that European countries with higher tobacco control efforts have reduced smoking prevalence and improved lung cancer mortality rates. It is predicted that the improved implementation of tobacco control policies could potentially prevent 1.65 million cases over a 20-year period across Europe [20].

1.2.3 Passive Smoking

While smoking is the biggest risk factor for developing lung cancer, up to 25% of cases worldwide occur in people who have never smoked [21]. Cases are also increasing in this group, rising from 8.9% of lung cancer diagnoses in 1990–1995, to 17% in 2011–2013 [22]. Risk factors other than smoking, e.g. exposure to radon and cooking smoke associated with biomass fuels are not exclusive to this group, implying there is heterogeneity in lung cancer aetiology.

Through passive smoking, non-smokers can be exposed to carcinogens and other substances found in cigarette smoke. However, trends in the incidence of lung cancer in this group are not well known because data on smoking status is only recently being collected by cancer registries. Meta-analyses have concluded there is approximately a 25% increased risk of lung cancer in never-smokers exposed to significant levels of second-hand smoke [23, 24].

1.2.4 E-Cigarettes

E-cigarettes and vaping have increased in use over the last few years. A heating coil is used to vaporise fluid containing nicotine and flavourings from a replaceable cartridge. The use of vaping varies, with some people employing E-cigarettes as a method of smoking cessation, some people using them alongside cigarettes, and others using them without a prior history of cigarette smoking. Forty percent of people aged 18–24 who vape were previously never-smokers [14], and 1 in 5 American high school students were current users of e-cigarettes in 2020 [25]. Vaping liquids contain a variety of substances, including both known and suspected carcinogens. Currently, long-term data are lacking regarding risk of lung cancer from e-cigarettes.

Heat not burn (HnB) tobacco is a product popular in East Asia, particularly Japan, and is now licenced in 30 countries. Tobacco is heated without combustion using an electronic element. Use has been increasing over recent years; in 2017 2.7% of people in Japan used HnB products [26], and 1.6% of American high school students engaged in this activity in 2020 [25]. HnB is purported as a safer nicotine delivery system, but there is a lack of independent evidence to support this claim, and the vast majority of research is sponsored by tobacco companies, which raises questions about potential bias in the methodology employed in the studies.

1.2.5 Air Pollution

Air pollution has wide geographical variation in both severity and constituents. A combination of vehicle emissions, industrial work and burning solid fuel contribute to pollution, with local practices and climate affecting both the severity of pollution and its constituent chemicals. Developing countries tend to have higher levels of pollution. This is at least partly attributable to the burning of biomass fuel in these countries [27]. Particulate matter (PM) is a key component of ambient air pollution. PM is a Group 1 carcinogen, with different size particles posing different risks. Small particles ($PM_{2.5}$) travel further into the lungs and contain a higher proportion of mutagenic substances, increasing the risk of lung cancer [28]. Three to 5% of lung cancer cases worldwide have been attributed to air pollution, with more than half of these in China and other East Asian countries [27].

1.2.6 Radon

Radon may account for up to 10% of lung cancer cases and is the most significant risk factor in never-smokers [22]. It is a radioactive gas produced as part of the natural breakdown of uranium from the soil. The breakdown of radon releases solid radioactive progeny, which can contribute to lung cancer risk through inhalation and adherence to the bronchial epithelium. While the highest concentrations of radon occur in areas of work underground (particularly uranium mines), air pollution with radon occurs in all settings. Outdoor levels tend to be low (5–15 Bq/m^3), but it can accumulate indoors, particularly in poorly ventilated rooms and basements [29]. Smoking increases the risks conferred by radon exposure. Estimates of the risk of developing lung cancer by age 75 at radon concentrations of 0, 100 and 400 Bq/m^3 for never-smokers are 0.4%, 0.5% and 0.7%, respectively, and 10%, 12% and 16% for smokers [30, 31].

1.2.7 Asbestos

Asbestos is a fibrous silicate material, which has been used in construction work since the nineteenth century and recognised as a harmful substance since the early 1900s. People who worked in construction (e.g. carpenters, plumbers and electricians), in shipyards and in the military are at high risk of exposure. There are six asbestos types: chrysolite (white asbestos), amosite (brown asbestos), crocidolite (blue asbestos), anthophyllite, tremolite and actinolite. Chrysolite is the most commonly used form, while tremolite and actinolite are not used commercially, but are found as contaminants in other products. It can be divided into two fibre types: serpentine has curly fibres and includes chrysolite, and amphibole (along with five other asbestos variants) has needle-like fibres [32].

Asbestos-related diseases include both malignant and non-malignant conditions affecting the lungs and pleura, and are caused by inhalation of asbestos fibres. Exposure to amphibole asbestos confers a greater risk of malignancy than serpentine, although both fibre types are hazardous. Asbestos causes the vast majority of cases of malignant mesothelioma, and it is also thought to cause 5%–10% of lung cancer cases worldwide [14]. It can lead to all histological subtypes of lung cancer and is indistinguishable from lung cancers of other etiology. It is generally agreed that lung cancer may be attributed to asbestos if there is a known significant exposure and at least 10 years between exposure and diagnosis [33]. There is some debate as to whether asbestosis (i.e. evidence of diffuse lung parenchymal disease) must be present for lung cancer to develop. Pleural plaques do not confer an increased lung cancer risk. It is unclear whether fibrosis is a prerequisite to developing lung cancer, or simply confers an additional risk [33].

The combined effects of asbestos exposure and smoking are synergistic rather than additive. While asbestos exposure increases lung cancer risk by fivefold, cigarette smoking remains a more potent risk factor, increasing risk by around tenfold. In a smoker, the cumulative risk of lung cancer following asbestos exposure is increased 50-fold [14, 33].

1.2.8   Infection

Chronic inflammation secondary to infections has been implicated in the formation of lung cancer. Of note, pulmonary tuberculosis (TB) has been shown to increase lung cancer risk. Although the worldwide incidence of TB is decreasing by approximately 2% a year, it continues to represent a significant burden of disease [14, 22].

HIV infection also increases the risk of lung cancer. It is the most common non-AIDS defining malignancy in HIV positive individuals. Although there is a high smoking prevalence among people with HIV, the relative risk of developing lung cancer is 2.5 regardless of smoking status [14].

1.2.9   Genetics and Family History

While environmental exposures are very important in the development of lung cancer, genetic factors also play a role. Fewer than 20% of smokers will eventually develop lung cancer, and cases can occur in never-smokers, indicating that other factors also contribute [34]. Owing to shared exposures in family members, determining the degree of genetic predisposition can be difficult; nevertheless, there is evidence of increased lung cancer risk in those with a family history of lung cancer, particularly for those diagnosed at a young age. Nearly 7% of lung cancer patients diagnosed prior to age 69 had a family history of lung cancer [35].

First degree family members are estimated to have a 2–3.5 times increased risk of developing lung cancer, although it should be noted that risk is increased by 1.75 times for spouses, suggesting that a portion of this risk is due to shared environmental exposures [36]. Risk is highest in siblings, regardless of smoking status [37]. The association is strongest in those who are younger at presentation, particularly in those aged less than 50 years [35, 37].

Many studies have attempted to identify genetic mutations associated with lung cancer. A meta-analysis concluded there are currently 22 genetic variants in 21 genes that are strongly associated with developing lung cancer. There is evidence of variation between different ethnicities, which may partially explain the racial variation in cases. Different cancer subtypes were also associated with different genetic variants [34]. Some genetic variants were only identified in patients with lung cancer who were also smokers, indicating there is likely to be a compound effect of smoking and genetics. This hypothesis is supported by the observation that there is an increased risk of lung cancer (1.51) in smokers with a family history of pulmonary malignancy compared to those without [37].

1.3 Conclusion

While multiple factors may contribute to the development of lung cancer, smoking is far and away the most important risk factor. Consequently, worldwide incidence varies in concert with the local smoking prevalence. In the West, lung cancer rates among men have declined since the 1980s, reflecting the decrease in smoking in this group approximately 20 years earlier. In women, lung cancer rates are only now reaching their peak, owing to the later decrease in smoking prevalence. As smoking rates continue to increase in less developed countries, we are likely to see an ongoing rise in lung cancer incidence in these regions. Although smoking contributes the greatest risk for lung cancer, never-smokers continue to develop this disease and pose an ongoing challenge as we try to eradicate this disease. The risk factors in this group are less well defined, and may be linked to genetic predisposition. Moving forward, establishing those at high risk of developing lung cancer and implementing tobacco control policies are essential to lung cancer care.

References

1. Cancer IAfRo. The Global Cancer Observatory—Lung 2021. https://gco.iarc.fr/today/data/factsheets/cancers/15-Lung-fact-sheet.pdf.
2. Peto R. Smoking, smoking cessation, and lung cancer in the UK since 1950: combination of national statistics with two case-control studies. BMJ. 2000;321(7257):323–9.
3. Thun M, Peto R, Boreham J, Lopez AD. Stages of the cigarette epidemic on entering its second century. Tob Control. 2012;21(2):96–101.
4. Sung H, Ferlay J, Siegel RL, Laversanne M, Soerjomataram I, Jemal A, et al. Global Cancer Statistics 2020: GLOBOCAN estimates of incidence and mortality worldwide for 36 cancers in 185 countries. CA Cancer J Clin. 2021;71(3):209–49.
5. UK CR. Lung cancer statistics. https://www.cancerresearchuk.org/health-professional/cancer-statistics/statistics-by-cancer-type/lung-cancer.
6. Barta JA, Powell CA, Wisnivesky JP. Global epidemiology of lung cancer. Ann Global Health. 2019;85(1):8.
7. Surveillance E, and End Results Program. Lung and bronchus long-term trends in SEER age-adjusted incidence rates, 1975-2018. 2021. https://seer.cancer.gov/explorer/application.html?site=47&data_type=1&graph_type=1&compareBy=sex&chk_sex_1=1&chk_sex_3=3&chk_sex_2=2&rate_type=2&race=1&age_range=1&hdn_stage=101&advopt_precision=1&advopt_show_ci=on&advopt_display=1.

8. Jani C, Marshall DC, Singh H, Goodall R, Shalhoub J, Al Omari O, et al. Lung cancer mortality in Europe and the United States between 2000 and 2017: an observational analysis. ERJ Open Res. 2021;7(4):00311-2021.

9. Allemani C, Matsuda T, Di Carlo V, Harewood R, Matz M, Nikšić M, et al. Global surveillance of trends in cancer survival 2000–14 (CONCORD-3): analysis of individual records for 37 513 025 patients diagnosed with one of 18 cancers from 322 population-based registries in 71 countries. Lancet. 2018;391(10125):1023–75.

10. Arnold M, Rutherford MJ, Bardot A, Ferlay J, Andersson TML, Myklebust TÅ, et al. Progress in cancer survival, mortality, and incidence in seven high-income countries 1995–2014 (ICBP SURVMARK-2): a population-based study. Lancet Oncol. 2019;20(11):1493–505.

11. England PH. Cancer survival in England: adult, stage at diagnosis, childhood and geographical patterns: NHS Digital. 2021. https://www.cancerdata.nhs.uk/survival/cancersurvivalengland.

12. Osmani L, Askin F, Gabrielson E, Li QK. Current WHO guidelines and the critical role of immunohistochemical markers in the subclassification of non-small cell lung carcinoma (NSCLC): moving from targeted therapy to immunotherapy. Semin Cancer Biol. 2018;52:103–9.

13. Lortet-Tieulent J, Soerjomataram I, Ferlay J, Rutherford M, Weiderpass E, Bray F. International trends in lung cancer incidence by histological subtype: adenocarcinoma stabilizing in men but still increasing in women. Lung Cancer. 2014;84(1):13–22.

14. De Groot PM, Wu CC, Carter BW, Munden RF. The epidemiology of lung cancer. Transl Lung Cancer Res. 2018;7(3):220–33.

15. Risch HA, Howe GR, Jain M, Burch JD, Holowaty EJ, Miller AB. Are female smokers at higher risk for lung cancer than male smokers? Am J Epidemiol. 1993;138(5):281–93.

16. Doll R, Hill AB. Smoking and carcinoma of the lung. BMJ. 1950;2(4682):739–48.

17. Kulhánová I, Forman D, Vignat J, Espina C, Brenner H, Storm HH, et al. Tobacco-related cancers in Europe: the scale of the epidemic in 2018. Eur J Cancer. 2020;139:27–36.

18. Prevention CfDCa. Cigarette smoking and tobacco use among people of low socioeconomic status | CDC; 2021.

19. Statistics OoN. Adult smoking habits in the UK: 2019. Cigarette smoking habits among adults in the UK, including the proportion of people who smoke, demographic breakdowns, changes over time and use of e-cigarettes; 2020.

20. Feliu A, Filippidis FT, Joossens L, Fong GT, Vardavas CI, Baena A, et al. Impact of tobacco control policies on smoking prevalence and quit ratios in 27 European Union countries from 2006 to 2014. Tob Control. 2019;28(1):101–9.

21. Chapman AM, Sun KY, Ruestow P, Cowan DM, Madl AK. Lung cancer mutation profile of EGFR, ALK, and KRAS: meta-analysis and comparison of never and ever smokers. Lung Cancer. 2016;102:122–34.

22. Corrales L, Rosell R, Cardona AF, Martín C, Zatarain-Barrón ZL, Arrieta O. Lung cancer in never smokers: the role of different risk factors other than tobacco smoking. Crit Rev Oncol Hematol. 2020;148:102895.

23. Kim A-S, Ko H-J, Kwon J-H, Lee J-M. Exposure to secondhand smoke and risk of cancer in never smokers: a meta-analysis of epidemiologic studies. Int J Environ Res Public Health. 2018;15(9):1981.

24. Taylor R, Najafi F, Dobson A. Meta-analysis of studies of passive smoking and lung cancer: effects of study type and continent. Int J Epidemiol. 2007;36(5):1048–59.

25. Gentzke AS, Wang TW, Jamal A, Park-Lee E, Ren C, Cullen KA, et al. Tobacco product use among middle and high school students—United States, 2020. MMWR. 2020;69(50):1881–8.

26. Simonavicius E, Mcneill A, Shahab L, Brose LS. Heat-not-burn tobacco products: a systematic literature review. Tob Control. 2019;28(5):582–94.

27. Cancer IAfRo. Air pollution and cancer. IARC Sci Publ. 2013;161.

28. Hamra GB, Guha N, Cohen A, Laden F, Raaschou-Nielsen O, Samet JM, et al. Outdoor particulate matter exposure and lung cancer: a systematic review and meta-analysis. Environ Health Perspect. 2014;122(9):906–11.

29. Organization WH. Radon and health 2021 [updated 02/02/2021]. https://www.who.int/news-room/fact-sheets/detail/radon-and-health.
30. Darby S, Hill D, Auvinen A, Barros-Dios JM, Baysson H, Bochicchio F, et al. Radon in homes and risk of lung cancer: collaborative analysis of individual data from 13 European case-control studies. BMJ. 2005;330(7485):223.
31. radiation Iagoi. Radon and public health. Public Health England; 2009.
32. center TM. Types of asbestos - chrysotile, actinolite, tremolite & more 2021. https://www.asbestos.com/asbestos/types/.
33. Klebe S, Leigh J, Henderson DW, Nurminen M. Asbestos, smoking and lung cancer: an update. Int J Environ Res Public Health. 2019;17(1):258.
34. Wang J, Liu Q, Yuan S, Xie W, Liu Y, Xiang Y, et al. Genetic predisposition to lung cancer: comprehensive literature integration, meta-analysis, and multiple evidence assessment of candidate-gene association studies. Sci Rep. 2017;7(1):8371.
35. Li X, Hemminki K. Inherited predisposition to early onset lung cancer according to histological type. Int J Cancer. 2004;112(3):451–7.
36. Jonsson S. Familial risk of lung carcinoma in the icelandic population. JAMA. 2004;292(24):2977.
37. Coté ML, Liu M, Bonassi S, Neri M, Schwartz AG, Christiani DC, et al. Increased risk of lung cancer in individuals with a family history of the disease: a pooled analysis from the International Lung Cancer Consortium. Eur J Cancer. 2012;48(13):1957–68.

Chapter 2
Health Disparities in Lung Cancer Screening

Katrina Steiling and Ariella Krones

2.1 Overview of Health Disparities in Lung Cancer

The first step to understanding how health disparities interact with LCS is to identify the existing disparities in lung cancer diagnosis, treatment, and mortality. Health disparities are defined as differences in health that are closely linked to social, economic, or environmental factors [1, 2]. Disparities in health can occur in relation to race and ethnicity, sex, gender and gender identity, mental health, disability, socioeconomic status, and geographical location [2]. Health disparities can also intersect across these dimensions.

Lung cancer rates are highest in individuals who are Black and in Native Hawaiians, with similar trends in lung cancer mortality [3]. In a 2020 Cancer Statistics assessment, lung cancer incidence in Non-Hispanic Black men was 82.7/100,000 versus 72.4/1000 in White men and lung cancer related mortality was 70.4/100,000 in Non-Hispanic Black men versus 51.8/100,000 for their White counterparts [4]. Lung cancer stage at diagnosis also varies by race, with 41% of lung cancers in Black individuals diagnosed at Stage IA as compared to 46% in White individuals. In addition to differences in stage at the time of diagnosis, surgical resection is less likely to be recommended to individuals who are Black with early-stage lung cancer compared to those that are White [5]. These observations suggest that racial differences in lung cancer mortality may be, in part, related to differences in cancer stage and treatment recommendations for early-stage disease.

In addition to racial disparities, there are other health disparities observed in lung cancer. While women have an overall lower risk of lung cancer than men [3], lung

K. Steiling (✉) · A. Krones
Section of Pulmonary, Allergy, and Critical Care Medicine, Boston University School of Medicine, Boston, MA, USA
e-mail: steiling@bu.edu

cancer rates are declining faster in men compared to women [6]. Women are also more likely to undergo limited resection for an early-stage lung cancer as compared to men [7]. Individuals with severe mental illness, such as schizophrenia, are at higher risk for death from lung cancer [8]. Large differences related to socioeconomic level have also been observed, with higher death rates from lung cancer occurring in men with lower attained education level [9]. Cigarette smoking, the leading cause of lung cancer, is similarly associated with income level, years of education, and insurance status [10].

Further research, however, is needed to determine if factors such as gender identity, geographic location, or disability status are associated with differences in lung cancer rates and outcomes.

2.2   The Landscape of Health Disparities in Lung Cancer Screening

The same disparities that affect lung cancer diagnosis rates and treatment modalities have affected the uptake and consistent use of LCS. These include different rates of LCS based on race and gender, location and environment, education level, and economic status or insurance type. While the relationship between some of these associations may appear more straightforward (e.g., lack of access to CT scanners and LCS programs in some rural areas), the associations and causative factors underlying them are often complex.

2.2.1   *Disparities Associated with Patient Demographics Including Race and Gender*

Rates of LCS have increased since its initial endorsement by the United States Preventive Services Task Force (USPSTF) and Centers for Medicare and Medicaid Services (CMS) [11–13] but remain quite low overall in the United States (US). In 2016, only 2% of eligible individuals underwent LCS [14]. This was assessed using data from the 2016 Lung Cancer Screening Registry. Lower rates of LCS have been observed in patients who are Black. Even when screening criteria are met, Black patients are less likely to utilize LCS. In a single center study, 37.6% of eligible Black patients were screened for lung cancer as compared to 46% of White patients [15]. In a survey on LCS rates in transgender versus cisgender individuals, transgender individuals while almost as equally likely to be eligible for LCS, were less likely to report having LCS (2.3% of transgender respondents versus 17.2% of cisgender respondents) [16]. Finally, patients with severe mental illness have delays associated with the diagnosis and treatment of lung cancer [17], with a standardized mortality rate of up to 2.2 [18]. Compounding these findings are data demonstrating that those with severe mental illness have at times a 1.13 times higher risk of delayed or no follow-up when enrolled in lung cancer screening [19]. These observations suggest that disparities in lung cancer screening may similarly affect this patient population.

Rates of adherence to continued annual LCS are similarly suboptimal [Fig. 2.1], with one meta-analysis suggesting that only 45% of patients with a negative or normal appearing initial LCS exam return for their annual follow-up imaging [12]. Notably, the range of adherence to annual screening in this study was between 8% and 86%, suggesting that there may be significant differences in completion of annual screening, which may vary by clinical setting or demographics. This finding has been supported by a study showing lower rates of completion for lung cancer screening follow-up exams in individuals who are Black, compared to those who are White [13].

Beyond disparities in LCS initiation and follow-up, there may be additional disparities in LCS eligibility criteria [Fig. 2.1]. USPSTF and CMS guidelines for LCS

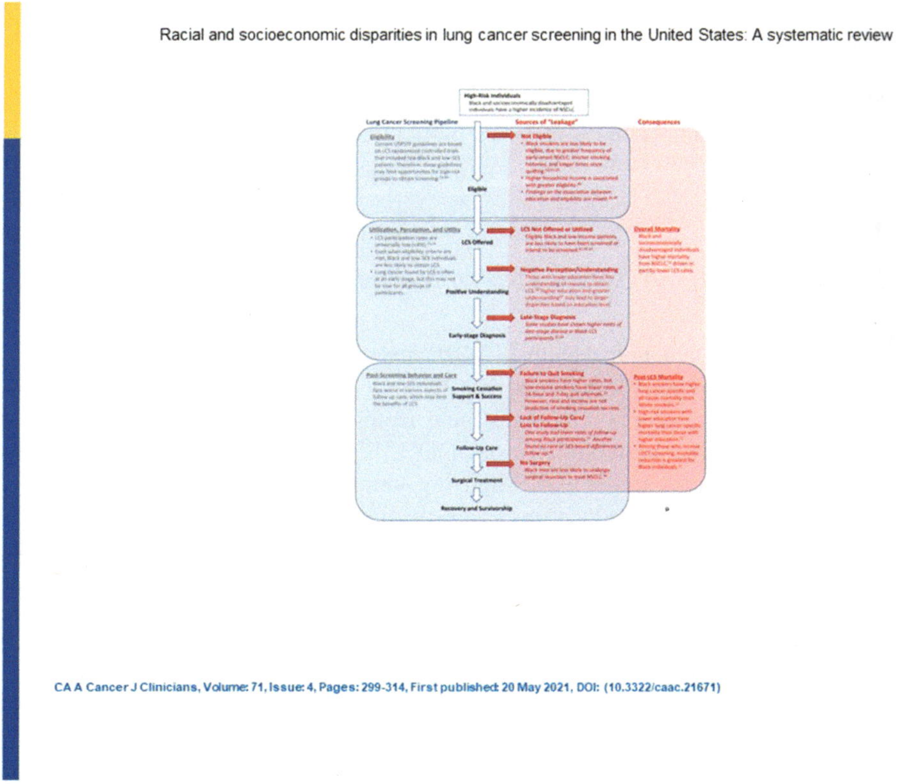

Racial and socioeconomic disparities in lung cancer screening in the United States: A systematic review

CA A Cancer J Clinicians, Volume: 71, Issue: 4, Pages: 299-314, First published: 20 May 2021, DOI: (10.3322/caac.21671)

Fig. 2.1 Lung cancer screening pipeline. This diagram shows findings related to racial and socioeconomic disparities in lung cancer screening that were captured by a systematic review. Statements in italics indicate contentious or ambiguous results. (Reprinted with permission from Wiley Publishing LLC)

are based primarily on age and smoking history [20, 21]. However, these guidelines do not account for differences seen in lung cancer risk and tobacco use patterns that are associated with race, ethnicity, socioeconomic status, and gender [22–24]. Earlier versions of the USPSTF LCS eligibility guidelines, which required higher cumulative cigarette smoke exposure (e.g., pack years), unintentionally resulted in racial disparities in screening eligibility. Specifically, African American individuals who smoke have higher rates of lung cancer despite lower reported pack years, and are also diagnosed with lung cancer at earlier ages compared to individuals who are White [22].

Several organizations have publicly recognized the bias in the initial sets of LCS eligibility criteria, including the USPSTF [21, 25, 26]. The USPSTF has since released updated guidance, lowering the age of onset of screening to 50 years and reducing the pack-year smoking history from 30 to 20 years, to reduce disparities in lung cancer screening eligibility [25]. However, it is unlikely that these modifications have eliminated disparities entirely [23]. Furthermore, while these guidelines will undoubtedly increase the volume of LCS examinations, in line with a national goal from the US Department of Health and Human Services [27], it is possible that increasing the overall rates of lung cancer screening without addressing underlying health inequities may ultimately and unintentionally exacerbate disparities exemplified by missed or delayed diagnostic follow-up testing [28]. Further research is needed to determine the optimal methods for providing LCS options and follow-up care to all populations equitably.

2.2.2 The Role of Social Determinants of Health (SDOH)

The social determinants of health (SDOH) are used to understand the various circumstances that impact individual and community health [29, 30], and thus can serve as a useful touchpoint to understand factors that contribute to disparities in LCS. There are five main domains of SDOH [Fig. 2.2]. The domain of economic stability encompasses access to safe housing, employment, and adequate health protections. The domain of education access includes the ability to learn and understand language in addition to health literacy and numeracy. The domain of health care access refers to the ability to engage with comprehensive health care on a regular basis, and to access reliable and affordable medical care. The domain of neighborhood and built environment consists of factors in the physical environment such as air quality, exposure to second-hand smoke, access to broadband, and the effects of systemic racism. Finally, the domain of social and community context encompasses general social support networks.

In the context of LCS, SDOH are associated with lower screening rates [Fig. 2.1]. Several studies suggest associations between the economic stability and health care access domains and LCS rates. Eligible patients with lower incomes are less likely to undergo LCS [15, 31]. Other studies have identified associations between neighborhood and built environment and rates of LCS. Utilization of LCS

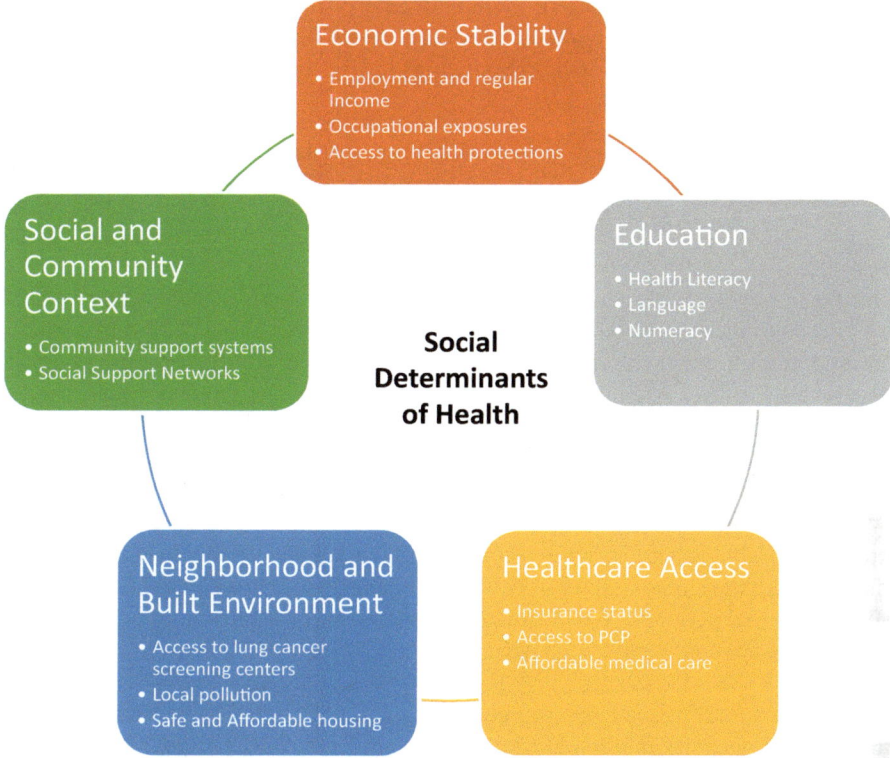

Fig. 2.2 Social determinants of health. This graph illustrates the five domains for social determinants of health. The five domains include economic stability, education access, health care access and quality, neighborhood and built environment, and social and community context

is lower among individuals that are uninsured [32] or who have government-based health insurance [31]. There is also marked geographic variation in LCS rates, with significantly lower rates of screening in the South and Southwest part of the US [33]. Individuals living in historically redlined neighborhoods, often urban areas, who identified as Black were less likely to undergo LCS [34]. Compounding low rates of LCS based on geographical location, awareness of LCS may be lower among individuals living in urban areas as compared to those living in suburban or rural areas [31].

2.3 Barriers to Lung Cancer Screening

While several demographic factors and SDOH are associated with lower LCS rates, this observation is likely to be related to multiple barriers to obtaining screening [Fig. 2.1]. These barriers can manifest at the level of health policy, the health care system, the individual patient, or the health care provider. These barriers, and the interaction between these barriers, may impede LCS across all populations with particular impacts on minoritized populations [24].

2.3.1 Barriers to Lung Cancer Screening That Act at the Health Policy Level

One barrier to equitable access to LCS lies in the limitations in developing eligibility criteria to identify patients that might benefit from screening. Eligibility criteria are important in order to select the highest risk patients and minimize the potential harms of LCS [20]. Although tobacco use is the major risk factor for lung cancer, current LCS eligibility guidelines do not account for other risk factors for lung cancer including air quality, environmental or occupational exposures, or family history. Current LCS eligibility guidelines are based on randomized clinical trials that defined risk for lung cancer by cumulative cigarette smoke exposure as measured by pack years. This approach, while accounting for the greatest source of lung cancer risk (tobacco use), may unintentionally bias against patients who have higher exposure to external pollution, environmental tobacco smoke exposure, or other occupational exposures such that they have an equivalent risk for lung cancer despite lower overall pack years [3, 22].

Another potential systemic source of bias in LCS eligibility guidelines are the low rates of diversity in clinical trial enrollment. Earlier LCS guidelines in the US were based on a randomized trial in which only ~4% of participants were Black [22, 29]. The largest European trial of LCS initially excluded women, but ultimately showed a greater benefit of screening in a small subgroup of women ultimately enrolled [35]. The lack of racial, ethnic, socioeconomic, and gender diversity in clinical trial participants may unintentionally bias eligibility criteria for LCS. This has been demonstrated in two studies showing that LCS guidelines based on the National Lung Screening Trial disproportionately exclude individuals who are Black and have higher lung cancer risk but lower reported pack years [22, 36].

2.3.2 Barriers to Lung Cancer Screening That Act at the Health System Level

Geographical location and lack of physical access to LCS may also be a barrier to screening for some patients. However, the data describing associations between urban and rural locations and completion of LCS is mixed and may instead suggest that other factors may interact with geography to influence screening rates. A single center study in Philadelphia showed that individuals who are Black had a lower rate of LCS, and that screening rates were even lower among Black individuals who lived in majority Black neighborhoods [11]. This suggests the potential for complex relationships between structural factors in the neighborhood and built environment and completion of LCS. Other data emphasize the risk of lower screening rates in rural populations.

In the US, there are marked differences in initial and annual LCS rates based on geographic region [33], with the highest screening rates in the Northeast and the lowest rates in the Western region. These geographical differences in screening rates correlate to numbers of physicians, rates of individuals with health insurance [14, 37], and availability of LCS facilities [34, 38, 39]. The differences in screening according to geographic location may be exacerbated not only by availability of screening facilities but also by the costs of traveling for the screening exam [37].

Lack of access to a primary care provider may also be a barrier to LCS. The Centers for Medicare and Medicaid Services (CMS) requires a shared decision-making visit to discuss the potential benefits and harms of screening prior to performing the LCS low-dose computed tomography scan [20]. This shared decision-making is often performed in the context of a primary care visit or during a discussion of routine health care maintenance. However, one-quarter of patients do not have a primary care provider [40], and this may limit access to and evaluation for LCS. Further exacerbating disparities in access to LCS is the observation that minorities, and patients without health insurance are less likely to have a regular source for medical care [40]. Future studies are needed to better understand the optimal approach to identify patients who are potentially eligible for LCS and connect them with a health care provider to discuss whether LCS is right for them.

2.3.3   Barriers to Lung Cancer Screening That Act at the Patient Level

While individual patients are certainly not the cause of low LCS rates, factors that act at the patient level, such as SDOH, may exacerbate inequities in LCS. Understanding these barriers might lead to better approaches to improve disparities in LCS. In addition to the association of lower rates of screening with race [15], income [15, 31, 41], and neighborhood or geographical location [11, 34, 42], access to health insurance and insurance status are also associated with lower LCS rates [31]. In a single center study conducted prior to standard insurance coverage of LCS exams, completion of annual LCS was significantly higher among individuals who received free screening, as compared to patients who were required to pay for the CT scan [43]. Participants in the self-pay group who did undergo annual LCS were more likely to be college educated, White, and perceived a higher cancer risk [43]. Another single center study found that patients with Medicaid had six times the odds of missing follow-up screening when compared to patients with private insurance [42]. These findings suggest that insurance coverage of LCS exams plays an important role in completion of screening for potentially eligible patients.

Patient language (English proficiency) and health literacy may additionally contribute to disparities in LCS. CMS requires the use of a decision aid during shared decision-making visits for LCS [20]. However, these materials are often not available in languages other than English, and frequently contain graphs and statistical explanations that may be challenging for patients to understand [44, 45]. In one study, patients with lower levels of education attainment had less understanding about why they were being screened [46]. A lack of understanding about the reasons for LCS may unintentionally lead to low rates of initial screening or completion of annual follow-up. There may be associations between the formal educational level attained and tobacco use that ultimately influence lung cancer risk [3, 22]. However, patients with lower levels of educational attainment are less likely to be eligible for LCS [47, 48], even though these patients may have an overall higher risk of lung cancer [48].

2.3.4   Barriers to Lung Cancer Screening That Act at the Health Care Provider Level

Several factors that act at the health care provider level might impact rates of LCS [49–51]. Many of these factors are practical barriers that may limit the ability of providers to offer screening. These include the lack of staff and clinic structure to identify eligible patients, ensure completion of annual screening exams, and manage abnormal screening findings such as incidental lung nodules or findings concerning for malignancy [50]. In one survey, 72% of respondents had a discussion about LCS with their doctor but tests were ordered in only 52% of patients [49]. While the source of this discrepancy is unclear, it suggests that factors related to clinical workflow management or health care provider knowledge about insurance coverage of LCS may be contributing. Automated systems for managing incidental pulmonary nodule detection may improve the rates of completion for follow-up imaging [52]. Similar approaches may have utility in tracking completion of annual lung cancer screening exams.

The time and expertise required to conduct a full shared decision-making conversation about LCS may also limit providers' ability to provide equitable care. Providers who serve patients with multiple health problems and/or limited access to regular health care may find that those patients have too many other acute medical concerns, limiting the available time to discuss health maintenance topics including LCS [37]. Qualitative content analysis of transcribed primary care visits for patients eligible for LCS suggests that the overall quality of shared decision-making is poor, with little discussion of the potential harms of screening [53]. Decision aids are also infrequently used in the shared decision-making discussions [53, 54], despite their required use by CMS. Prior to February of 2022, CMS required an in-person shared decision-making visit prior to LCS. CMS has since updated their requirements to allow telehealth visits for counseling and shared decision-making. Studies have suggested that conducting the shared decision-making discussion via telephone may decrease barriers to LCS [55, 56].

Another potential provider-level barrier to LCS may be an incomplete understanding of LCS guidelines compounded by nuances in the primary data from which these guidelines are derived [57]. In one survey, a total of 87.9% of primary care providers reported that low-dose computed tomography was useful for LCS in people who used tobacco, but, in contrast to eligibility guidelines, 40% reported that it was also helpful in non-smokers [49]. Similarly, 36.8% of respondents reported that chest radiography was also helpful [49], even though this method does not have utility for LCS [58]. These misunderstandings of guidelines for LCS have implications for clinical practice that may contribute to low LCS rates. For example, while current guidelines recommend low-dose computed tomography for LCS [20, 21], only 52% of survey respondents ordered a low-dose CT scan, whereas 43.1% ordered a chest X-ray for screening [49]. Improving health care provider education about LCS guidelines and eligible patient populations may help improve LCS rates.

There is also the potential for implicit bias to influence recommendations for LCS. Implicit bias refers to unconscious attitudes that nevertheless impact behavior [59] and can be measured by the implicit association test [60]. Implicit bias in the context of LCS may relate to demographic factors, SDOH, or stigma related to tobacco use. However, the potential role of implicit bias in lung cancer screening rates is unclear and requires further study.

2.4   Overcoming Disparities in Lung Cancer Screening

There are promising approaches to overcoming barriers to lung cancer screening and reducing health disparities, but these interventions have not been studied systematically or on a large scale. Interventions that might reduce barriers to lung cancer screening and address disparities in screening range from changes at the health policy level to improve equity in clinical trials and standardized data collection and reporting, to improved insurance coverage for screening examinations through programs such as Medicaid expansion, to improved access to screening centers for populations most affected by lung cancer [23]. Innovative solutions to geographic barriers, such as mobile screening units [61], may in fact be a key step in broadening the health system to reach more patients.

Patient navigation is a promising approach to address barriers to screening that act at the patient level. Patient navigators connect patients to community resources and assist them in accessing complex health systems [62]. This intervention has been shown to be effective in improving access to and diagnostic resolution of other cancer screening exams [63, 64]. The observation that patients with Medicaid or housing insecurity were more likely to miss appointments for LCS [42] suggests that patient navigation may be an effective intervention to improve completion of LCS.

Interventions that have the potential to improve barriers to lung cancer screening at the provider level include resources aimed at improving provider education about lung cancer screening, support for shared decision-making visits, and support for integrating discussions about lung cancer screening into busy clinical schedules [23]. The potential role for implicit bias reduction training and culturally sensitive communication techniques are also areas for future study [55, 56].

In summary, while overall lung cancer screening rates remain low for all eligible patients, lower rates of initial screening and screening follow-up are associated with race, gender, severe mental illness, socioeconomic status, and geographic factors. Barriers to lung cancer screening act at multiple intersecting spheres, including at the level of health policy, the health system, the individual patient, and the health care providers. The causative factors underlying the barriers to lung cancer screening are complex and may interact across multiple different levels. The full promise of low-dose computed tomography screening for lung cancer screening as a method for reducing individual and population-level lung cancer mortality cannot be realized until the health care disparities affecting screening rates are addressed.

References

1. Disparities | healthy people 2020. [Cited 2022 Jan 28]. https://www.healthypeople.gov/2020/about/foundation-health-measures/Disparities.
2. HHS action plan to reduce racial and ethnic health disparities. https://www.minorityhealth.hhs.gov/assets/pdf/hhs/HHS_Plan_complete.pdf.
3. Stram DO, Park SL, Haiman CA, Murphy SE, Patel Y, Hecht SS, et al. Racial/ethnic differences in lung cancer incidence in the multiethnic cohort study: an update. J Natl Cancer Inst. 2019;111(8):811.
4. Siegel RL, Miller KD, Jemal A. Cancer statistics, 2020. CA Cancer J Clin. 2020;70(1):7–30.
5. Soneji S, Tanner NT, Silvestri GA, Lathan CS, Black W. Racial and ethnic disparities in early-stage lung cancer survival. Chest. 2017;152(3):587–97.
6. Jemal A, Miller KD, Ma J, Siegel RL, Fedewa SA, Islami F, et al. Higher lung cancer incidence in young women than young men in the United States. N Engl J Med. 2018;378(21):1999–2009.
7. Balekian AA, Wisnivesky JP, Gould MK. Surgical disparities among patients with stage I lung cancer in the National Lung Screening Trial. Chest. 2019;155(1):44–52.
8. Bradford DW, Goulet J, Hunt M, Cunningham NC, Hoff R. A cohort study of mortality in individuals with and without schizophrenia after diagnosis of lung cancer. J Clin Psychiatry. 2016;77(12):e1626–30.
9. Siegel R, Ward E, Brawley O, Jemal A. Cancer statistics, 2011. CA Cancer J Clin. 2011;61(4):212–36.
10. Delva J, Tellez M, Finlayson TL, Gretebeck KA, Siefert K, Williams DR, et al. Cigarette smoking among low-income African Americans: a serious public health problem. Am J Prev Med. 2005;29(3):218–20.
11. Lake M, Shusted CS, Juon HS, McIntire RK, Zeigler-Johnson C, Evans NR, et al. Black patients referred to a lung cancer screening program experience lower rates of screening and longer time to follow-up. BMC Cancer. 2020;20(1):561.
12. Lin Y, Fu M, Ding R, Inoue K, Jeon CY, Hsu W, et al. Patient adherence to lung CT screening reporting & data system-recommended screening intervals in the United States: a systematic review and meta-analysis. J Thorac Oncol. 2022;17(1):38–55.

13. Kunitomo Y, Bade B, Gunderson CG, Akgün KM, Brackett A, Cain H, et al. Racial differences in adherence to lung cancer screening follow-up: a systematic review and meta-analysis. Chest. 2022;161(1):266–75.
14. Pham D, Bhandari S, Pinkston C, Oechsli M, Kloecker G. Lung cancer screening registry reveals low-dose CT screening remains heavily underutilized. Clin Lung Cancer. 2020;21(3):e206–11.
15. Steiling K, Loui T, Asokan S, Nims S, Moreira P, Rebello A, et al. Age, race, and income are associated with lower screening rates at a safety net hospital. Ann Thorac Surg. 2020;109(5):1544–50.
16. Stowell JT, Parikh Y, Tilson K, Narayan AK. Lung cancer screening eligibility and utilization among transgender patients: an analysis of the 2017-2018 United States behavioral risk factor surveillance system survey. Nicotine Tob Res. 2020;22(12):2164–9.
17. Flores EJ, Park ER, Irwin KE. Improving lung cancer screening access for individuals with serious mental illness. J Am Coll Radiol. 2019;16(4 Pt B):596–600.
18. Tran E, Rouillon F, Loze JY, Casadebaig F, Philippe A, Vitry F, et al. Cancer mortality in patients with schizophrenia. Cancer. 2009;115(15):3555–62.
19. Núñez ER, Caverly TJ, Zhang S, Glickman ME, Qian SX, Boudreau JH, et al. Adherence to follow-up testing recommendations in US veterans screened for lung cancer, 2015-2019. JAMA Netw Open. 2021;4(7):e2116233.
20. NCA—screening for lung cancer with low dose computed tomography (LDCT) (CAG-00439N)—decision memo. [Cited 2022 Jan 28]. https://www.cms.gov/medicare-coverage-database/view/ncacal-decision-memo.aspx?proposed=N&NCAId=274.
21. Krist AH, Davidson KW, Mangione CM, Barry MJ, Cabana M, Caughey AB, et al. Screening for lung cancer: US preventive services task force recommendation statement. J Am Med Assoc. 2021;325(10):962–70.
22. Aldrich MC, Mercaldo SF, Sandler KL, Blot WJ, Grogan EL, Blume JD. Evaluation of USPSTF lung cancer screening guidelines among African American adult smokers. JAMA Oncol. 2019;5(9):1318–24.
23. Patricia Rivera M, Aldrich MC, Henderson LM, Cardarelli R, Carter-Harris L, Crothers K, et al. Addressing disparities in lung cancer screening eligibility and healthcare access. An official American Thoracic Society statement. Am J Respir Crit Care Med. 2020;202(7):E95–112.
24. Sosa E, D'Souza G, Akhtar A, Sur M, Love K, Duffels J, et al. Racial and socioeconomic disparities in lung cancer screening in the United States: a systematic review. CA Cancer J Clin. 2021;71(4):299–314.
25. Davidson KW, Mangione CM, Barry MJ, Cabana MD, Caughey AB, Davis EM, et al. Actions to transform US preventive services task force methods to mitigate systemic racism in clinical preventive services. JAMA. 2021;326(23):2405–11.
26. Lin JS, Hoffman L, Bean SI, O'Connor EA, Martin AM, Iacocca MO, et al. Addressing racism in preventive services: methods report to support the US Preventive Services Task Force. J Am Med Assoc. 2021;326(23):2412–20.
27. Increase the proportion of adults who get screened for lung cancer—C-03—healthy people 2030 | health.gov. [Cited 2021 Dec 17]. https://health.gov/healthypeople/objectives-and-data/browse-objectives/cancer/increase-proportion-adults-who-get-screened-lung-cancer-c-03.
28. Horn DM, Haas JS. Expanded lung and colorectal cancer screening—ensuring equity and safety under new guidelines. N Engl J Med. 2022;386(2):100–2. https://doi.org/10.1056/NEJMp2113332.
29. Sources for data on SDOH | social determinants of health | CDC. [Cited 2021 Dec 6]. https://www.cdc.gov/socialdeterminants/data/index.htm.
30. Social determinants of health (SDOH). [Cited 2021 Dec 6]. https://catalyst.nejm.org/doi/full/10.1056/CAT.17.0312.
31. Carter-Harris L, Slaven JE, Monahan PO, Shedd-Steele R, Hanna N, Rawl SM. Understanding lung cancer screening behavior: racial, gender, and geographic differences among Indiana long-term smokers. Prev Med Rep. 2018;10:49–54.

32. Zahnd WE, Eberth JM. Lung cancer screening utilization: a behavioral risk factor surveillance system analysis. Am J Prev Med. 2019;57(2):250–5.
33. Okereke IC, Nishi S, Zhou J, Goodwin JS. Trends in lung cancer screening in the United States, 2016-2017. J Thorac Dis. 2019;11(3):873–81.
34. Poulson MR, Kenzik KM, Singh S, Pavesi F, Steiling K, Litle VR, et al. Redlining, structural racism, and lung cancer screening disparities. J Thorac Cardiovasc Surg. 2022;163(6):1920–1930.e2.
35. de Koning HJ, van der Aalst CM, de Jong PA, Scholten ET, Nackaerts K, Heuvelmans MA, et al. Reduced lung-cancer mortality with volume CT screening in a randomized trial. N Engl J Med. 2020;382(6):503–13.
36. Fiscella K, Winters P, Farah S, Sanders M, Mohile SG. Do lung cancer eligibility criteria align with risk among Blacks and Hispanics? PLoS One. 2015;10(11):e0143789.
37. Wang GX, Baggett TP, Pandharipande PV, Park ER, Fintelmann FJ, Percac-Lima S, et al. Barriers to lung cancer screening engagement from the patient and provider perspective. Radiology. 2019;290(2):278–87.
38. Kale MS, Wisnivesky J, Taioli E, Liu B. The landscape of US lung cancer screening services. Chest. 2019;155(5):900–7.
39. Tailor TD, Choudhury KR, Tong BC, Christensen JD, Sosa JA, Rubin GD. Geographic access to CT for lung cancer screening: a census tract-level analysis of cigarette smoking in the United States and driving distance to a CT facility. J Am Coll Radiol. 2019;16(1):15–23.
40. Levine DM, Linder JA, Landon BE. Characteristics of Americans with primary care and changes over time, 2002-2015. JAMA Intern Med. 2020;180(3):463–6.
41. Japuntich SJ, Krieger NH, Salvas AL, Carey MP. Racial disparities in lung cancer screening: an exploratory investigation. J Natl Med Assoc. 2018;110(5):424–7.
42. Shin D, Fishman MDC, Ngo M, Wang J, LeBedis CA. The impact of social determinants of health on lung cancer screening utilization. J Am Coll Radiol. 2022;19(1 Pt B):122–30.
43. Wildstein KA, Faustini Y, Yip R, Henschke CI, Ostroff JS. Longitudinal predictors of adherence to annual follow-up in a lung cancer screening programme. J Med Screen. 2011;18:154–9.
44. Haas K, Brillante C, Sharp L, Elzokaky AK, Pasquinelli M, Feldman L, et al. Lung cancer screening: assessment of health literacy and readability of online educational resources. BMC Public Health. 2018;18(1):1356.
45. Gagne SM, Fintelmann FJ, Flores EJ, McDermott S, Mendoza DP, Petranovic M, et al. Evaluation of the informational content and readability of US Lung Cancer Screening Program Websites. JAMA Netw Open. 2020;3(1):e1920431.
46. Hall DL, Lennes IT, Carr A, Eusebio JR, Yeh GY, Park ER. Lung cancer screening uncertainty among patients undergoing LDCT. Am J Health Behav. 2018;42(1):69–76.
47. Li CC, Matthews AK, Rywant MM, Hallgren E, Shah RC. Racial disparities in eligibility for low-dose computed tomography lung cancer screening among older adults with a history of smoking. Cancer Causes Control. 2019;30(3):235–40.
48. Han SS, Chow E, Ten Haaf K, Toumazis I, Cao P, Bastani M, et al. Disparities of national lung cancer screening guidelines in the US population. JNCI J Natl Cancer Inst. 2020;112(11):1136.
49. Raz DJ, Wu GX, Consunji M, Nelson R, Sun C, Erhunmwunsee L, et al. Perceptions and utilization of lung cancer screening among primary care physicians. J Thorac Oncol. 2016;11(11):1856–62.
50. Simmons VN, Gray JE, Schabath MB, Wilson LE, Quinn GP. High-risk community and primary care providers knowledge about and barriers to low-dose computed topography lung cancer screening. Lung Cancer. 2017;106:42–9.
51. Triplette M, Kross EK, Mann BA, Elmore JG, Slatore CG, Shahrir S, et al. An assessment of primary care and pulmonary provider perspectives on lung cancer screening. Ann Am Thorac Soc. 2018;15(1):69–75.
52. Singh H, Koster M, Jani C, Rupal A, Walker A, Khoory J, et al. Nodule net: a centralized prospective lung nodule tracking and safety-net program. Respir Med. 2022;192:106737.
53. Brenner AT, Malo TL, Margolis M, Elston Lafata J, James S, Vu MB, et al. Evaluating shared decision making for lung cancer screening. JAMA Intern Med. 2018;178(10):1311–6.

54. Nishi SPE, Lowenstein LM, Mendoza TR, Lopez Olivo MA, Crocker LC, Sepucha K, et al. Shared decision-making for lung cancer screening: how well are we "sharing"? Chest. 2021;160(1):330–40.
55. Tanner NT, Banas E, Yeager D, Dai L, Hughes Halbert C, Silvestri GA. In-person and telephonic shared decision-making visits for people considering lung cancer screening: an assessment of decision quality. Chest. 2019;155(1):236–8.
56. Fagan HB, Fournakis NA, Jurkovitz C, Petrich AM, Zhang Z, Katurakes N, et al. Telephone-based shared decision-making for lung cancer screening in primary care. J Cancer Educ. 2020;35(4):766–73.
57. Khairy M, Duong DK, Shariff-Marco S, Cheng I, Jain J, Balakrishnan A, et al. An analysis of lung cancer screening beliefs and practice patterns for community providers compared to academic providers. Cancer Control. 2018;25(1):1073274818806900.
58. Oken MM, Hocking WG, Kvale PA, Andriole GL, Buys SS, Church TR, et al. Screening by chest radiograph and lung cancer mortality: the prostate, lung, colorectal, and ovarian (PLCO) randomized trial. JAMA. 2011;306(17):1865–73.
59. Maina IW, Belton TD, Ginzberg S, Singh A, Johnson TJ. A decade of studying implicit racial/ethnic bias in healthcare providers using the implicit association test. Soc Sci Med. 2018;199:219–29.
60. Greenwald AG, McGhee DE, Schwartz JLK. Measuring individual differences in implicit cognition: the implicit association test. J Pers Soc Psychol. 1998;74(6):1464–80.
61. Crosbie PA, Balata H, Evison M, Atack M, Bayliss-Brideaux V, Colligan D, et al. Implementing lung cancer screening: baseline results from a community-based 'lung health check' pilot in deprived areas of Manchester. Thorax. 2019;74(4):405–9.
62. Meade CD, Wells KJ, Arevalo M, Calcano ER, Rivera M, Sarmiento Y, et al. Lay navigator model for impacting cancer health disparities. J Cancer Educ. 2014;29(3):449–57.
63. Paskett ED, Katz ML, Post DM, Pennell ML, Young GS, Seiber EE, et al. The Ohio Patient Navigation Research Program: does the American Cancer Society patient navigation model improve time to resolution in patients with abnormal screening tests? Cancer Epidemiol Biomark Prev. 2012;21(10):1620–8.
64. Freund KM, Battaglia TA, Calhoun E, Darnell JS, Dudley DJ, Fiscella K, et al. Article impact of patient navigation on timely cancer care: the Patient Navigation Research Program. J Natl Cancer Inst. 2014;106(6):dju115.

Chapter 3
Best Practices in Lung Cancer Screening

Carey C. Thomson, Humberto Choi, Jorge Ataucuri-Vargas, Peter Mazzone, Jonathan Li, Andrea B. McKee, and Teresa Giamboy

C. C. Thomson (✉)
Multidisciplinary Thoracic Oncology and Lung Cancer Screening Program, Pulmonary and Critical Care Division, Mt Auburn Hospital/Beth Israel Lahey Health, Harvard Medical School, Cambridge, MA, USA
e-mail: cthomson@mah.harvard.edu

H. Choi · J. Ataucuri-Vargas
Department of Pulmonary Medicine, Thoracic Oncology Program for the Respiratory Institute and Lung Cancer Screening Program, Cleveland Clinic, Cleveland, OH, USA

P. Mazzone
Lung Cancer Program for the Respiratory Institute and the Lung Cancer Screening Program, Cleveland Clinic, Cleveland, OH, USA

J. Li
Primary Care, Department of Medicine, Beth Israel Deaconess Medical Center, Harvard Medical School, Boston, MA, USA

A. B. McKee
Radiation Oncology, Lahey Hospital and Medical Center, Tufts University School of Medicine, Boston, MA, USA

T. Giamboy
Lung Cancer Screening Program, Jefferson Health, Philadelphia, PA, USA

© The Author(s), under exclusive license to Springer Nature Switzerland AG 2022
J. V. Baptiste et al. (eds.), *Lung Cancer Screening*,
https://doi.org/10.1007/978-3-031-10662-0_3

3.1 Evidence Base for Lung Cancer Screening

Humberto Choi, Jorge Ataucuri-Vargas and Peter Mazzone

3.1.1 Introduction

Lung cancer screening (LCS) is the application of a test in asymptomatic individuals at risk of developing lung cancer with the goal of detecting lung cancer at an early stage. The outcome of successful screening is a reduction in lung cancer mortality. Several screening tests have been evaluated to date. Early research evaluated chest radiography (CXR) and sputum cytology as potential screening tests [1–3]. Advances in computed tomography (CT) scanning techniques led to improved sensitivity in detecting small suspicious tumors, paving the way for the evaluation of low-dose CT scan (LDCT) as a screening test.

We will discuss the evidence base for the benefits and harms of screening, including studies investigating sputum cytology and chest radiography, followed by LDCT observational and randomized clinical trials, and finally evidence related to shared decision-making, cost-effectiveness, smoking cessation, and non-lung nodule findings.

3.1.2 Measuring Benefits and Harms of Screening

An ideal cancer screening test should be readily available, inexpensive, acceptable to those being screened, and carry little risk from its performance. The test should detect cancer in a localized state with high sensitivity, while detecting little pseudodisease, leading to minimal harms from the evaluation of screen-detected findings [4]. There should be evidence that treatment of the cancer is more successful when detected at an early stage.

The benefit of cancer screening can be expressed as the absolute risk reduction (ARR), relative risk reduction (RRR), or number needed to screen (NNS) to prevent adverse outcomes (e.g., mortality) [5].

Cancer-specific mortality reduction is the ideal outcome when evaluating the efficacy of a screening test. Other outcomes reported include cancer detection rates, stage shift, stage at detection, survival, and overall mortality.

The use of survival as a surrogate of screening test efficacy is discouraged due to the influence of lead-time bias (early detection of asymptomatic cancer lengthens the time a patient is aware of the disease without affecting mortality), length-time bias (the detection of a disproportionate number of indolent cancers through screening), and overdiagnosis bias on the interpretation of the findings [4].

Potential screening harms include: (1) complications from the performance of the screening test (e.g., radiation-associated malignancy), (2) false-positive results with ensuing physical harms from their evaluation and psychological repercussions, (3) over-detection and ensuing overtreatment of cancers that would not have impacted well-being, and (4) avoidable costs related to screening (to the individual or society, real or opportunity costs) [5].

3.1.3 Screening Modalities

3.1.3.1 Chest Radiography and Sputum Cytology

The first tests assessed for LCS were CXR and sputum cytology. In the late 1960s the National Cancer Institute formed a task force known as the Cooperative Early Lung Cancer Group, leading to several randomized clinical trials assessing the efficacy of CXR and sputum cytology for LCS. These randomized controlled trials included: Johns Hopkins study, Memorial Sloan-Kettering Study, and the Mayo Lung Project. In these trials, all individuals were above 45 years of age with a smoking history. Participants were randomized to screening with a CXR at various intervals versus the combination of a CXR and sputum cytology. The Johns Hopkins study enrolled 10,386 individuals with an 8-year follow-up. The Memorial Sloan-Kettering Study enrolled 10,040 male participants with a 5- to 8-year follow-up. The Mayo Lung Project enrolled 10,933 male outpatients who underwent a baseline CXR and sputum cytology before randomization with a 5-year follow-up. Survival and lung cancer mortality rates were similar in both control and intervention arms, except in the Mayo Clinic study, where 5-year survival was higher in the screening group (40%) vs. the control group (15%). Sputum cytology failed to show efficacy as an LCS tool [3, 6, 7]. The lack of a true control arm in these studies complicated their interpretation.

The role of CXR as an LCS modality was more definitively assessed in the Prostate, Lung, Colorectal, and Ovarian (PLCO) cancer randomized trial. The study enrolled 154,901 participants aged 55–74 years, from 1993 to 2001. The intervention group received an annual CXR for 4 years while the control group received usual medical care. Lung cancer incidence (per 10,000 person-years), followed through 13 years, was 20.1 in the intervention group and 19.2 in the usual care group. Lung cancer mortality was similar between groups. Thus, LCS with annual CXR was not able to show a reduction in lung cancer mortality [8].

The studies described above represent the early search for effective LCS modalities. Unfortunately, none of the trials were able to show a reduction in lung cancer mortality, despite improved survival.

3.1.3.2 Low-Dose CT Scan

Observational Studies

The early LDCT screening studies were observational cohort studies from the United States and Japan (Table 3.1). The Early Lung Cancer Action Project (ELCAP) was an observational single-center cohort study. One thousand asymptomatic volunteers, above 60 years, with at least 10 pack-years of cigarette use, who were fit to undergo surgical resection were enrolled from 1993 through 1998. A LDCT scan and CXR

Table 3.1 Low-dose CT scan observational studies

Study	Year/location	Sample size (number of enrolled patients)	Inclusion criteria		Outcome	Screening methods	Screened lung cancer detection rate at baseline	Stage I	Survival rate
			Age	Smoking history (PYH = pack-years smoking history)					
ELCAP*	1992/USA	1000	>60 years old; >10 PYH		Nodule	LDCT	2.70%	85%	–
					Malignancy detection	CXR	0.70%	57%	
I-ELCAP+	1993/USA, Europe, China, Israel, Japan	31,567	>40 years old with current/prior/second-hand smoking, (16% never-smokers)		10-year lung cancer-specific survival	LDCT	1.28%	85%	80% (10-year)
ALCA++	1993/Japan	1611	40–75 years old; (14% never-smokers)		Screen detected lung cancer, survival rate	LDCT	0.81%	78.6%	71% (5-year)
						CXR	0.31%		
						Sputum cytology	0.25%		
Sone et al. [9]	1996/Japan	5480	40–74 years old; (55.4% never-smokers)		10-year survival	LDCT	1.04% (baseline and repeat LDCT screening)	83%	86.2% (10-year)
			10% <50 years old			Sputum cytology	0.02%		

*Early Lung Cancer Action Project. +International Early Lung Cancer Action Project. ++ Anti-Lung Cancer Association project

Pts patients, LDCT low-dose CT scan, CXR chest radiography

was performed in each study subject at baseline. Nodule detection, malignancy rate and stage were assessed. Baseline LDCT identified lung cancer in 2.7% of study subjects while 0.7% of study subjects had lung cancer detected by baseline CXR. Twenty-six of the 27 lung cancers detected by baseline LDCT were resectable [10].

The International ELCAP (I-ELCAP) study was a multicenter cohort study that significantly expanded the findings of the ELCAP study, enrolling 31,567 asymptomatic individuals from 1993 through 2005 at least 40 years of age, with elevated lung cancer risk based on smoking history, second-hand smoke exposure, and occupational exposure (asbestos, beryllium, uranium, and radon). A baseline LDCT scan was performed in each enrolled individual, followed by a total of 27,456 annual LDCT screenings. The primary outcome was 10-year lung cancer-specific survival in those with stage I lung cancer detected by LDCT scan. Of the 484 participants who received a diagnosis of lung cancer, 85% had clinical stage I lung cancer. In this subgroup, the estimated 10-year survival rate was 88% [11]. As a reference, the largest US cancer registry in 2003, the National Cancer Institute's Surveillance, Epidemiology, and End Results (SEER) registry, reported an 8-year survival rate of 75% among patients with pathological stage I cancer who had undergone resection [12].

Both ELCAP and I-ELCAP studies showed screened-detected lung cancers were predominantly detected at an early stage by LDCT scans showing higher survival rates compared to national registries.

A population-based LDCT screening study from Japan enrolled 5480 participants (55.4% were never-smokers). A baseline LDCT scan was obtained in 1996 followed by repeat LDCT screening in 1997–1998. Lung cancer (80.7% stage I) was detected in 63 individuals (57 lung cancer cases were detected by LDCT). The 10-year lung cancer-specific survival was 86.2% [9].

The Anti-Lung Cancer Association (ALCA) is an observational study that enrolled 1682 participants into a single arm. Every 6 months, LDCTs, CXRs, and sputum cytology were performed on each participant. Of the 14 lung cancers detected at initial screening, 57% were detected by LDCT scan alone, 10% by LDCT scan and CXR, 7% by sputum cytology, and 21% by all 3 methods. Eighty-one percent of cancers detected were stage I. The 5-year survival rate for screen-detected lung cancer was 76.2% [13].

These observational studies provided early evidence of the potential efficacy of LDCT for lung cancer screening. LDCT showed a higher lung cancer detection rate than CXR and sputum cytology and the ability to detect early-stage disease. Due to the observational nature of these studies, they were unable to assess lung cancer mortality reduction as an outcome.

3.1.3.3   Randomized Clinical Trials

National Lung Screening Trial

The National Cancer Institute (NCI) sponsored the National Lung Screening Trial (NLST), a landmark randomized controlled clinical trial that enrolled 53,454 patients between 2002 and 2004. Thirty-three United States medical centers participated. The aim was to determine if screening a high-risk population with a LDCT could reduce lung cancer-specific mortality compared to screening with a CXR. The population included current or former smokers ages 55–74 with at least 30 pack-years of smoking and having smoked within the past 15 years. Three annual rounds of screening LDCT or CXR were performed with a median follow-up of 6.5 years [14].

Adherence to the 3-year screening protocol was 95% in the LDCT group compared to 93% in the CXR group. Up to 39.1% of the participants in the former group versus 16.0% of the latter group had at least one positive screening result (lung nodule 4 mm or larger). There were 247 deaths from lung cancer per 100,000 person-years of follow-up in the LDCT arm versus 309 per 100,000 person-years after screening with CXR. This corresponds to a lung cancer-specific mortality risk reduction of 20% favoring the LDCT group.

Overall mortality was 6.7% lower in the LDCT group (1877 deaths) compared to the CXR group (2000 deaths). Lung cancer incidence was higher and more lung cancers were detected at an early stage in the LDCT group (1060 lung cancers, 50% stage I) compared to the patients who underwent screening with CXR (941 lung cancers, 31.1% stage I). The number needed to screen with LDCT to prevent 1 death from lung cancer was 320 (at 6.5 years of follow-up) and 303 at 12.3 years of extended follow-up [15]. A NLST posthoc analysis showed black individuals derived the most benefit of lung cancer mortality reduction [16].

The NLST was the first randomized clinical trial showing a significant reduction in lung cancer mortality using LDCT compared to CXR. These results led to sweeping changes in professional organization clinical guidelines, practice parameters, and insurance coverage. The implementation of national LDCT screening based on the NLST eligibility criteria could avoid 18,000 premature deaths annually [17, 18]. ·

European Randomized Lung Cancer Screening Trials

Along with the NLST, several randomized clinical trials were performed in Europe, including the NELSON trial which will be discussed in a separate section. Seven trials in Europe enrolled 36,000 participants using LDCT as the screening intervention and usual care (no screening) as the control [19]. As a group, these trials are known as the European randomized lung cancer screening trials (EUCT).

The aim was to combine their data once a minimum of 170,300 person-years follow-up were reached in the control arm. This would achieve 90% power to demonstrate a lung cancer mortality reduction of at least 25% depending on lung cancer risk, compliance, and contamination rates [20]. ·

The European randomized clinical trials include: NELSON = Dutch–Belgian lung cancer screening trial (Nederlands–Leuvens Longkanker Screenings Onderzoek), DANTE = (Detection and screening of early lung cancer with Novel imaging Technology) trial, DLCST = Danish Lung Cancer Screening Trial, ITALUNG = Italian Lung Cancer Screening Trial, MILD = Multicentric Italian Lung Detection, UKLS = UK Lung Cancer Screening, and LUSI = German Lung Cancer Screening Intervention Trial.

Table 3.2 Low-dose CT scan randomized clinical trials

Study	Location	Enrolled patients (screening/control arm)	Age (years)	Smoking history PY = pack-year smoking history	Follow-up duration	Screening interval and duration	Baseline description of positive nodules: positive (+), negative (–)
NLST	United States	26,722 (LDCT) 26,732 (CXR)	55–74	current or former smokers >30PY, quit <15 years	6.5 years (extension to 12.3 years)	Three annual screens	(+) non–calcified nodule ≥4mm, adenopathy, effusion (–) nodule <4mm
NELSON	Netherlands, Belgium	7915 (LDCT) 7907 (no screening)	50–74	current or former smokers >15PY, quit <10 years	10 years	Four screening rounds: interval after baseline: 1, 2, and 2.5 years	(+) solid >500mm³, pleural based > 10mm or VDT <400 days on 3 month CT scan (–) <50 mm3or VDT > 600 days
DANTE	Italy	1264 (LDCT) 1186 (yearly clinical review)	60–74 (men only)	current or former smokers >20 PY, quit <10 years	4 years	Five annual screens	(+) smooth solid ≥ 10mm, spiculated solid ≥6mm; GGO ≥ 10mm. (–) ≤5mm smooth or calcified solid
DLCST	Denmark	2052 (LDCT) 2052 (no screening)	50–70	current or former smokers >20PY, quit <10 years	10 years	Five annual screens	(+) >15mm or with suspicious morphology (–) <5mm or benign characteristics
ITALUNG	Italy	1613 (LDCT) 1593 (no screening)	55–69	current or former smokers >20 PY, quit <10 years	7 years	Four annual screens	(+) solid ≥5mm, nonsolid ≥10mm (–) solid <5mm, nonsolid <10mm
MILD	Italy	1190 (annual LDCT) 1186 (biennial LDCT) 1723 (no screening)	49–75	current or former smokers >20 PY, quit <10 years	10 years	Five annual screens and three biennial screens combined	(+) >250 mm³ (–) < 60 mm³
UKLS	United Kingdom	2000 (LDCT) 2000 (no screening)	50–75	5% risk of lung cancer in 5 years	10 years	One screen	(+) 500 mm³, pleural based > 10mm or VDT < 400 days (–) <15mm³, pleural based ≤3mm
LUSI	Germany	2029 (LDCT) 2023 (no screening)	50–69	current or former smokers >15 PY, quit <10 years	8.89 years	Five annuals screens	(+) >10 mm or VDT ≤400 days (–) <5mm or VDT >600 days

NLST National Lung Screening trial, *NELSON* Dutch–Belgian lung-cancer screening trial (Nederlands–Leuvens Longkanker Screenings Onderzoek), *DANTE* (Detection And screening of early lung cancer with Novel imaging TEchnology) trial, *DLCST* Danish Lung Cancer Screening Trial, *ITALUNG* Italian Lung Cancer Screening Trial, *MILD* Multicentric Italian Lung Detection, *UKLS* UK Lung Cancer Screening, *LUSI* German Lung Cancer Screening Intervention Trial, *LDCT* Low-dose CT scan, *CXR* chest radiography, *VDT* volume-doubling time, *GGO* ground-glass opacity

The EUCT share in common a LDCT screening group compared with a no-screening arm, and enrolling only high-risk individuals who currently or previously smoked. Nodule-volume management protocols were used in NELSON, DLCST, LUSI, and UKLS [21–24].

The EUCT study designs differed from the NLST in study eligibility criteria, recruitment methods, control group interventions, method for assessment of nodules, definition of a positive scan and screening scan intervals (Table 3.2) [25].

Taken in isolation most of the EUCT trials, except the NELSON trial, did not show a difference in lung cancer mortality in the LDCT arm compared to the control arm, though they were not powered to do so [19].

Some salient features of the EUCT include: The MILD trial suggested equal sensitivity, specificity, positive predictive value (PPV), and negative predictive value (NPV) of annual versus biennial LDCT screening [26]. The German Lung cancer Screening Intervention (LUSI) found a lung cancer mortality reduction among the women who underwent LDCT [23]. The UK Lung Cancer screening trial (UKLS) used a risk-based prediction model to select participants (the Liverpool Lung Project risk model version 2) and endorsed CT volumetry-based management protocols for lung nodules discovered during screening [24].

NELSON Trial

The Dutch–Belgian lung cancer screening trial (Nederlands–Leuvens Longkanker Screenings Onderzoek [NELSON]) was a European population-based, randomized, controlled trial initiated in 2000. Its aim was to determine if LDCT screening could lead to a reduction in lung cancer mortality. The trial enrolled 15,792 participants (84% men) aged 50–75 years old, currently or previously smoked [quit ≤10 years ago] who had smoked >15 cigarettes a day for >25 years or >10 cigarettes a day for >30 years [27, 28]. The screening group underwent 4 LDCT screening rounds at intervals of 1, 2, and 2.5 years while the control group received no screening (usual care). Volume and growth-based nodule management protocols were used to determine nodule management plans. A positive test result was defined as a nodule volume above >500 mm^3 or volume-doubling time lower than 400 days (as assessed on a 3-month follow-up scan for nodules 50–500 mm^3) (Table 3.3).

In the male cohort, 9.2% of the LDCT scans resulted in an indeterminate result (nodule 50–500 mm^3) leading to a repeat CT scan to calculate volume-doubling time before a final test screening outcome could be labeled. In follow-up rounds, 55% of new nodules were resolved. Finally, 2.1% of LDCT scans were test-positive requiring further workup leading to 203 screen-detected lung cancers (58.6% stage IA or IB, 52% adenocarcinoma subtype). The positive predictive value was 43.8%. The overdiagnosis rate was 8.9%.

Table 3.3 Population characteristics, nodule management, and screening intervals in NLST compared to NELSON trial

	NLST	NELSON trial
Eligibility criteria		
Age (years)	55–74	50–74
Smoking status (PY = pack-year smoking history)	Current or former smokers >30 PY, quit <15 years	Smokers >15 cigarettes/day for >25 years or >10 cigarettes/day >30 years, quit <10 years
Male (%)	59	83.5
Screening interval	Three annual screens	Four screening rounds: interval after baseline: 1, 2, and 2.5 years
Nodule assessment	2D caliper measurement	3D volumetric analysis
Nodule management	+: (+) non-calcified nodule ≥4 mm, adenopathy, effusion	+: (partial) solid nodules volume >500 or 50–500 mm^3 with VDT[a] <400 days on 3-month repeat CT scan
Positive nodule		
Follow-up (years)	6.5 years (planned)/12.3[b] years (extension)	10
Number needed to screen	320[c]/303[b]	133

NLST National Lung Screening Trial, *NELSON* Dutch–Belgian lung cancer screening trial (Nederlands–Leuvens Longkanker Screenings Onderzoek)
[a] Volume-doubling time
[b] Extended follow-up
[c] Based on planned median 6.5-year follow-up. [c] Calculated on an extended follow-up (12 years) [15]

At 10-year follow-up, lung cancer mortality in the screened group was reduced by 24% in men and 33% in women compared to the control group. There was no difference in the overall mortality, although the study was not powered to assess this specific outcome [29]. A higher lung cancer mortality reduction was found in women compared to men, but lower representation in the population enrolled (16% were women) meant the study was not powered to detect a significant difference in women.

The NELSON trial is the second well-powered trial, preceded by the NLST, to have confirmed lung cancer mortality reduction in high-risk patients undergoing lung cancer screening with LDCT scan.

3.1.4 Patient Selection

Optimal patient selection maximizes lung cancer screening benefits and reduces potential harms. Mirroring the inclusion criteria of the NLST was an initial framework for LCS patient selection. Several professional organizations recommended LCS based on the NLST eligibility criteria (Table 3.4). However, the population enrolled in the NLST, compared to a 2002–2004 U.S. Census survey of tobacco use who met the NLST eligibility criteria, were younger, had a higher level of education, and were more likely to be former smokers. Minority populations were underrepresented, 4.4% were black, and 1.7% were Hispanic/Latino [18]. In their study, Pinksy et al. showed that among individuals being diagnosed with lung cancer only 27% will be eligible for LCS under the NLST enrolment criteria [30]. These limitations on the NLST eligibility criteria led to the National Comprehensive Cancer Network (NCCN) and American Association of Thoracic Surgery (AATS) guidelines to include additional risk factors associated with lung cancer to define high-risk groups who will benefit from LCS with LDCT. Several risk prediction models were also developed to assess lung cancer risk (e.g., Prostate, Lung, Colorectal, and Ovarian [PLCO$_{2012}$] model).

A systematic review of randomized clinical trials (including the NELSON trial and NLST) and modeling studies led the United States Preventive Services Task Force (USPSTF) to expand the recommended LCS eligibility criteria. The modeling studies were commissioned to the Cancer Intervention and Surveillance Modeling Network (CISNET) to determine the optimal eligibility screening age range, screening interval, benefits and harms of different screening strategies, including risk factor-based strategies (e.g., age, pack-year smoking history) compared with modified versions of multivariate risk prediction models [31].

The updated USPSTF recommended eligibility criteria include those adults aged 50–80 years who have a 20 pack-year smoking history and currently smoke or have quit within the past 15 years [32]. This update will increase the number of screening-eligible individuals by around 86% overall, and by 77% in non-Hispanic whites and non-Hispanic blacks, compared with the 2014 USPSTF recommended LCS criteria [33, 34].

Table 3.4 Professional societies recommendations on lung cancer screening

	Age (years)	Smoking history (pack-years)	Smoking cessation	Screening interval	Additional recommendations
USPSTF (2021)	50–80	≥20	<15 years	Annual	Screening should be discontinued once a person has not smoked for 15 years or develops a health problem that substantially limits life expectancy or the ability or willingness to have curative lung surgery.
ACCP (2021)	50–80	≥20	<15 years	Annual	Suggestion to use validated clinical risk prediction calculators, life expectancy estimates, or life-year gained calculations to assess net benefit for those outside the eligibility criteria based on age and smoking history
CMS (2014)[a]	55–77	≥30	<15 years	Annual	Shared decision-making visit required
NCCN (2019)[a]	55–74	≥30	<15 years	Annual	20 pack-years, age >50, and additional risk factors
ACS (2013)[a]	55–74	≥30	<15 years	Annual	
AATS (2012)[a]	55–79	≥30		Annual	20 pack-years, age >50 years, and risk ≥5% over 5 years
	50–79	>20			

ACCP American College of Chest Physicians, *ACS* American Cancer Society, *ASCO* American Society of Clinical Oncology, *CMS* Center for Medicaid & Medicare Services, *NCCN* National Comprehensive Cancer Network, *USPSTF* United States Preventative Services Task Force, *AATS* American Association of Thoracic Surgery
[a] Recommendations currently under revision

Screening should be discontinued once a person has not smoked for 15 years or develops a health problem that substantially limits life expectancy or the ability or willingness to have curative lung surgery [32]. The operational definition of the number or severity of medical comorbidities that will lead to an unfavorable balance of benefits and potential harms can be difficult to define on an individual level [35, 36].

Others have evaluated the use of lung cancer risk or LCS benefit prediction calculators to identify those who should be considered screen eligible [37, 38]. The updated American College of Chest Physicians (ACCP) lung cancer screening guideline suggests the use of validated clinical risk prediction calculators (e.g., Lung Cancer Death Risk Assessment Tool [LCDRAT]; PLCOM$_{2012}$ calculator; Bach calculator) and life expectancy estimates, or life-year gained calculators (e.g., Life Years Gained From Screening-CT (LYFS-CT) calculator) to assess those individuals with a high net benefit in order to offer annual lung cancer screening with LDCT [39].

3.1.5   Evidence of Potential Harms

Potential harms from lung cancer screening are a result of the performance of the test and/or the management of screen-detected findings. The management of screen-detected lung nodules leads to the greatest potential for harm. Other potential harms include the impact of cumulative radiation exposure, overdiagnosis, false positives, and their psychological burden.

There is substantial debate about the potential risk for radiation-associated malignancy related to radiation exposure from LCS with LDCT scans. Many estimates have been developed with varying results. In one study, the estimate for lifetime excess relative risk from radiation-associated lung cancer due to annual LDCT scans was calculated. In a 50-year-old female who smokes, the lifetime excess relative risk was 0.85%, and the excess risk in a 50-year-old male who smokes was 0.23% [40].

Overdiagnosis refers to the identification of a screen-detected lung cancer that would not have led to symptoms or harm in the individual [41]. This can occur because the identified cancer is quite indolent or because the individual has substantial comorbidities that lead to their death before cancer would have. In the NLST the estimate of overdiagnosis was 18.5%. On an extended follow-up to 11.3 years the estimate dropped to 3.1% [15]. A metanalysis based on 2 LCS randomized clinical trials with a low risk of bias found that 49% of screen-detected lung cancers were overdiagnosed [42]. If individuals with more severe comorbidities are enrolled in screening in practice the impact of overdiagnosis could be higher.

False-positive results in LCS can lead to further testing including invasive procedures. A study found the range of false positive rates among LCS studies was 7.9–49.3% for baseline screening. The variation was due to different definitions of positive results (e.g., nodule size thresholds) and different nodule management protocols (diameter-based and volumetric-based) [34]. The false positive rates tend to decrease with subsequent screening rounds. The false positive rate in the NLST (diameter-based nodule management protocol) was approximately 27% in each of the first 2 rounds, decreasing to 16.8% in the third round [28]. The false positive rate in the NELSON trial (volumetric-based nodule management protocol) was 19.8% at baseline, dropping to 7.1% at year 1, 9.0% for males at year 3, and 3.9% for males at year 5.5 of screening.

In the NLST, reported positive results led to invasive studies in 1.7% of those screened. Complications among screened individuals were reported in 0.1% [14, 43] A study estimated 23.4% of all invasive procedures for false positives would be prevented by using the Lung-RADS criteria [44].

Lung cancer screening has the potential to cause short-term psychological burden in individuals with an indeterminate scan result, although the adverse effects do not appear to persist long-term (>6 months) [45].

3.1.6 Shared Decision-Making Evidence in Lung Cancer Screening

A shared decision-making (SDM) visit provides an opportunity to discuss benefits along with the potential harms and uncertainties regarding LCS [35, 38, 46]. The Centers for Medicare and Medicaid Services (CMS) mandate a patient counseling and SDM visit before a patient undergoes LDCT screening [47]. The elements of a SDM visit include determination of patient eligibility criteria; information of LCS benefits and harms including use of decision aids; communication about the importance of LCS annual adherence, and smoking cessation counseling.

The quality of the SDM visit is highly variable. A recent cross-sectional study with 266 LCS participants found up to a third (33.6%) of patients have some decisional conflict regarding screening [48]. A total of 41.4% of patients answered LCS knowledge questions correctly. Lower knowledge levels were found in non-white and lower literacy patients. Overall, there is low use (30.7%) of educational materials and decision aids. Although most patients (66.3%) correctly identified smoking abstinence as the most effective method to lower lung cancer risk, almost a third of patients indicated that screening rather than smoking abstinence was the best way to lower the likelihood of lung cancer mortality. Another study found there is a decrease in knowledge retention regarding LCS benefits and harms 1 month after the SDM visit but remained higher than pre-SDM visit levels [49]. Both participants and providers tend to overestimate benefits and underestimate harms across studies [48, 50, 51].

3.1.7 Cost-Effectiveness of Lung Cancer Screening

The updated 2021 USPSTF lung cancer screening recommendations were analyzed in a cost-effectiveness study using a comparative modeling approach. Four independently developed and validated microsimulation models from the CISNET Lung Working Group were used to assess population-level health benefits and costs. The updated 2021 USPSTF LCS eligibility criteria were compared to 6 alternative criteria including the prior 2013 USPSTF LCS eligibility criteria. The willingness-to-pay threshold of $100,000 per quality-adjusted life-year (QALY) was used to define a strategy as cost-effective. The 2021 USPSTF LCS recommendations were found to be cost-effective compared to the prior 2013 USPSTF recommendations. The cost-effectiveness was found to be higher in women and with the formal inclusion of life expectancy in the eligibility criteria [52].

3.1.8 Smoking and Lung Cancer Screening

Smoking is the most important modifiable risk factor associated with the risk of developing lung cancer. Participation in LDCT screening provides an opportunity to offer tobacco treatment. Smoking cessation interventions are an essential component of a lung cancer screening program [38]. However, the outcome of smoking cessation in lung cancer screening settings have varied [53, 54].

Smoking cessation programs incorporated in LDCT screening can result in high smoking cessation rates (30%) [55]. The smoking habits analyzed in the NELSON and DLCST trials did not differ between the control and intervention arm but the abstinence rate was higher (17%) compared to the general population rate without smoking cessation interventions (3–7%) [54, 56, 57]. In a posthoc analysis of the NLST cohort, false-positive results reported to individuals who currently smoke and those who recently quit were associated with higher rates of abstinence both in the LDCT and the CXR arm. The abstinence rate achieved a plateau despite repeated reports of positive screening results. Conversely, negative imaging results reported to individuals who stopped smoking had high motivation rates for maintaining smoking abstinence. Of notice, those individuals who received a false-positive result had unchanged levels of relapse on a 5-year follow-up [58].

3.1.9 Non-lung nodule Findings

The rate of non-lung nodule findings depends on how a positive result is defined. When defined liberally, up to 94% of LDCT scans identify a non-lung nodule abnormal finding [59]. Non-lung nodule findings include: atherosclerosis (coronary artery calcium), thoracic aortic aneurysms, emphysema, pulmonary fibrosis, osteopenia/osteoporosis, thyroid, adrenal, hepatic, and renal nodules/masses, adenopathy, mediastinal lesions, and pleural disease.

The most frequent non-nodule findings are found in the respiratory (emphysema) and cardiovascular systems (coronary calcification). Most of the findings are not actionable, but a significant minority require specialty consultation (15%) and further testing (13%). Serious non-lung cancer findings such as triple-vessel coronary artery disease (CAD) and cancers of other organs can be identified. For example, 20.5% of patients with significant coronary artery calcification discovered during LCS had a change in management (mainly medical management and stress testing) [60].

Each program should establish who should be responsible for the management of non-lung nodule findings found in LCS, based on published guidelines [38, 61].

3.1.10 Evidence Needs

Despite the confirmed benefits of LDCT as an effective tool in lung cancer screening, there are still areas that would benefit from additional evidence. The optimal approach to the selection of those at risk and the processes of screening, such as the best way to do a SDM visit, how to incorporate smoking cessation in LCS, and how to ensure compliance with follow-up and annual screening. Further research is also needed in how to minimize disparities, how to provide access to screening and high-quality nodule management for the underinsured and those in rural locations.

The identification of patients with non-smoking risk factors (e.g., radon exposure, family history, occupational exposure, biomass fuels, second-hand smoke exposure, pulmonary fibrosis) who will benefit from LCS is still under study. A predictive model was developed that included patients who never smoked: $PLCO_{all2014}$ [62]. The calculated risk of patients who never smoked was below the threshold where screening would potentially have more benefits than potential harms regardless of the presence of other risk factors [62].

Potential adjunctive tools for optimization of LDCT screening in the future include the implementation of artificial intelligence (AI) and radiomics. A study using AI showed a decrease by 11% in false positives and by 5% in false negatives in a cohort [63–65]. Advances in the use of ultra-low-dose CT screening could potentially allow for a lower risk of radiation-associated malignancy [66].

3.1.11   Conclusion

Low-dose CT-based screening has been shown to reduce lung cancer mortality in individuals at high risk for developing lung cancer. Understanding the evidence that supports the benefit of screening and identifies potential harms from screening will assist with the implementation of high-quality screening in clinical practice.

3.2   Quality Indicators in Lung Cancer Screening Programs

Jonathan Li and Carey C. Thomson

Healthcare quality measures are standards for measuring the performance of healthcare providers to care for patients and populations. At a local level, adopting standardized quality measures is important in cancer screening programs in order to determine the reach and effectiveness of the program. It enables programs to track performance over time, and benchmark against peers or industry standards, and allows for the evaluation of success or lack thereof of local quality improvement initiatives. On a national level, this allows us to better understand trends, disparities, and enable comparison between disparate regions or health systems. Importantly, as healthcare payment systems shift from fee-for-service to value-based payment models, coordinated through accountable care organizations, having uniformly defined quality measures allows inclusion of these screening programs into incentive-based quality contracts between payers and care organizations to improve the quality of care for patients.

3.2.1 Challenges in Developing Quality Metrics in Lung Cancer Screening

The Healthcare Effectiveness Data and Information Set (HEDIS) is a tool developed through the National Committee for Quality Assurance (NCQA) to set standard definitions for healthcare performance measures. This is the most widely used set of performance measurement definitions in the managed care industry in the United States. While colorectal, breast, and cervical cancer screening measures are included in HEDIS—and thus are widely adopted quality measurements in value-based contracts across the United States—lung cancer screening is not [67]. There are multiple reasons for this. A significant challenge in measuring lung cancer screening rate (i.e., proportion of eligible population that is screened via low-dose CT scan) is that the population denominator is predicated upon having accurate data about patient smoking history (both the number of pack-years ever smoked, and time relative to quit date if applicable) which is heterogeneously obtained and documented in electronic medical records. In comparison, the other three aforementioned cancer screening measures in HEDIS are based solely on age threshold and gender (for breast and cervical cancer), without a further qualifier. Any attempt to measure lung cancer screening rates in a health system in the absence of reliable, patient-level smoking history data would be misleading. Currently there is no consensus among national experts that lung cancer screening should be included as a standard quality measure in HEDIS. While proponents argue that this would incentivize more comprehensive discussions and documentation about smoking histories, and therefore increase the eligible screening population, there are concerns that the nuances of shared decision-making, particularly with respect to the harms of over-testing, would be overshadowed by accountability to such a performance metric [68]. Even so, the discussion is moving in favor of developing a HEDIS measure to improve uptake of lung cancer screening.

3.2.2 Expert Consensus in Measuring Program Quality in Lung Cancer Screening

Though these challenges exist, there is a substantial opportunity to develop standardized quality metrics in lung cancer screening to both identify eligible populations, and to evaluate program quality for screened patients as it relates to appropriate follow-up completion. Developing a structure that supports evaluation and reporting of process, access, and quality metrics is essential. This is discussed more in Sect. 3.3. Lung cancer screening programs should regularly evaluate their program and its outcomes. The most comprehensive expert consensus on both of these needs is from the Implementation Strategies Task Group (ISTG) of the National Lung

Cancer Roundtable. The multidisciplinary ISTG reviewed existing evidence and practice, in keeping with process standards for quality metric development by the NCQA, to develop consensus on reasonable quality indicators related to processes and outcomes of chest CT lung cancer screening. Through this formal multi-step process, this group identified six lung cancer screening quality indicators that achieved expert consensus [69]:

1. Screening Appropriateness: The percentage of individuals who complete low-dose CT (LDCT) screening for lung cancer who are screening eligible based on United States Preventive Service Task Force (USPSTF) criteria.
2. Smoking Cessation: The percentage of people who currently smoke who participate in LDCT scan screening who have documentation of a smoking cessation intervention.
3. Compliance with Follow-up Recommendations Lung-RADS 1/2: The percentage of lung cancer LDCT scan screening-eligible individuals who completed an LDCT scan examination and are identified as having Lung CT Screening Reporting and Data System (Lung-RADS) category 1 or 2 findings who completed the next annual LDCT screening examination.
4. Compliance with Follow-up Recommendations Lung-RADS 3: The percentage of individuals who completed an LDCT scan lung cancer screening examination and were identified as having a Lung-RADS category 3 nodule in which surveillance LDCT scan is performed at 6 months (±2 months).
5. Compliance with Follow-up Recommendations Lung-RADS 4: The percentage of individuals who completed an LDCT scan lung cancer screening examination and were identified as having a Lung-RADS category 4 nodule in which a surveillance LDCT scan is performed at 3 months (±6 weeks) or additional diagnostic evaluation is performed within 3 months.
6. Evaluation of Concerning Findings: The time in days from identification of a Lung-RADS category 4B or 4X lung nodule or mass on an LDCT scan screening examination in someone with lung cancer, to the diagnosis of lung cancer.

In order to measure these six quality metrics for lung cancer screening, there must be a population health management system in place locally. This health management system should support the development of patient registries to easily identify eligible patients, and track patients as they progress through the program. Existing low-dose CT lung cancer screening programs may effectively partner with local population health management resources to provide data management and outreach capabilities for this population, to both expand the eligible population being screened and also reduce leakage ("loss to follow-up") of successfully screened patients who need ongoing screening or surveillance. Adoption of standard quality metrics for both screening rate and follow-up completion will allow assessment of performance trends locally, regionally, nationally, and by payor, and ultimately help to drive improvements in patient care.

3.2.3 National Trends in Screening Rates, Disparities, and Targets

The National Cancer Institute *Cancer Trends Progress Report* aims to quantify the progress made to reduce cancer mortality through research and healthcare delivery improvement. Lung cancer is one of five cancers measured and reported on. This report estimates national lung cancer screening rates per 2013 USPSTF guidelines through the National Health Interview Survey, a large, national, in-person survey conducted from 2010 to 2015 by the CDC. There are important limitations in this methodology as patients surveyed may overestimate or underestimate their lifetime smoking history, and may not know whether a CT chest scan was for screening or diagnostic purposes (both are included in the rate calculation), but this is accepted as the best national data currently available on lung cancer screening rates.

Based upon this survey, the most recent estimate (2015) is that 4.5% (95% CI 2.8–7.2) of eligible US adults were screened for lung cancer using a CT scan in the prior year. There were significant disparities by race. Non-Hispanic white persons were screened at a rate of 4.9% (3.0–8.0), while non-Hispanic Black persons had a rate of 1.7% (95% CI 0.6–5.0), and Hispanic persons a rate of 0.7% (95% CI 0.1–4.6) [70]. Through the Healthy People 2030 Initiative led by the U.S. Department of Health and Human Services, the goal is to increase this rate for all US adults to 7.5% by 2030 [71]. Achieving such an ambitious target requires attention at a local level to quality metrics which accurately quantify the eligible population and nudges providers to have more shared decision-making conversations with their patients about the important role of CT lung cancer screening.

3.3 Structure and Governance

Andrea McKee and Carey C. Thomson

Development of a Multidisciplinary Steering Committee can serve as a powerful coalition to guide program development, provide a forum to establish consensus, and promote a team-based approach to overcome obstacles to program implementation [72].

3.3.1 Steering Committee Governance of CT Lung Screening Programs

Change is hard; and the more people required to make a change, the harder it is to bring about. Lung cancer screening (LCS) program development is a team sport, with no one individual discipline able to do it alone. Steering Committees should be

Table 3.5 Lahey Hospital and Medical Center CT Lung Screening Program Mission

Save lives through early detection of lung cancer with responsible CT lung screening
Encourage the government to establish reimbursement for responsible CT lung screening
Encourage other centers of excellence in the treatment of lung cancer to offer responsible free CT lung screening until CMS establishes reimbursement
Break down prejudice faced by those at risk for lung cancer
Raise public awareness of the power of responsible CT lung screening to save lives
Provide a platform to explore relevant research questions

multidisciplinary and include clinicians, administrators, and staff from the departments of internal medicine, pulmonary, pathology, radiation and medical oncology, thoracic surgery, and radiology. This structure has been widely supported by leading organizations and specialty societies [72].

Steering committee members should be engaged specifically for their known ability to advocate for patients, develop programs, and for their political prowess to support implementation. Establishing a guiding mission can support the development of a successful program and process for LCS. To accomplish the mission requires a powerful coalition to guide program development, provide a forum to establish consensus, and work in concert to overcome obstacles to program implementation. The following mission from the Lahey Hospital and Medical Center (LHMC) Rescue Lung Rescue Life LCS program was developed prior to program implementation and serves as an example of such a mission [73] (Table 3.5):

3.3.2 Program Design

The steering committee should establish the program structure [72]. The structure of a screening program will depend on the type of institution, available resources, population, and the extent and breadth of the screening program. In many instances, lung cancer screening programs are embedded in pre-existing lung cancer and lung nodule clinics. The steering committee will evaluate the best "fit" for their institution.

Lung cancer screening programs may be centralized, decentralized, or combine components of centralized and decentralized models into a hybrid structure according to which staff will be responsible for managing the participants and data associated with the program [73]. Centralized programs require providers to refer their patients to a program where program staff conduct the SDM visit, order the LCS CT, follow and often manage the results of the study, and track quality and outcome metrics of the program. Decentralized programs are specifically designed to cost-effectively overcome the barriers to SDM without restricting access to screening [73, 74]. Primary Care Providers (PCPs) are preventive care experts best positioned to engage their patients in the shared decision-making (SDM) process for all screening decisions. To support their SDM process, LCS programs should ensure that PCPs and patients are aware of the criteria, risks, and benefits of LCS and of the process necessary to obtain a LCS study and manage the findings. Hybrid programs often rely on providers to conduct the SDM visit and order the study, but the program staff follow results and track program and participant data and metrics.

Patients and providers should be provided with decision aids in the form of written, electronic, and verbal communications. They should have access by telephone, email, and electronic medical record (EMR) to knowledgeable program personnel at multiple time points prior to enrollment. Data associated with program participants, the program process and outcomes, should be collected and evaluated to ensure high-quality LCS and management.

3.3.3 Provider Continuing Education

Prior to implementation of a LCS program, the steering committee should conduct an extensive continuing medical education campaign for local provider groups. For a successful program, this will require multiple face-to-face meetings between providers and program content experts, both within and outside the health system, to ensure that providers are well versed in their role in the SDM process. Provider directed literature should be developed by the multidisciplinary steering committee and sent to every referring provider inquiring about patient eligibility. The literature should include facts about the evidence base for lung cancer screening, program eligibility requirements, proven and theoretical risks of screening, mechanics of the CT screening process including how to order the exam, and descriptions of available smoking cessation resources. Programs should assess the feasibility of implementing a Best Practice Alert within the electronic health record to help providers identify the high-risk screening-eligible population. Face to face meetings with the primary care groups should continue at regular intervals to ensure ongoing engagement, as well as subsequent to any significant event in the realm of lung cancer screening. Individual score cards of a provider's performance are also useful for providers to compare their screening metrics to averages across the provider base in the following areas: *Number referred, number qualified, cancer detection rate and stages of those detected, smoking cessation rate, and medical record numbers of those they referred for screening who never presented for the exam* [73].

3.3.4 Community Outreach

Community outreach centered around small group meetings can also be an effective strategy for enhanced participation in lung cancer screening. Steering committee members can provide presentations at regional councils on aging, veteran's groups, military bases, professional firefighters associations, semi-professional sporting events, rotary clubs, chambers of commerce, health fairs, cancer walks, and lung advocacy events. These community education outreach campaigns in neutral settings, outside the clinical office or hospital environment, can raise awareness about the risks and benefits of screening in the patient's home environment among family and friends and further support the SDM process by facilitating conversations with "trusted others [75]."

3.3.5   Measuring Outcomes

Similar to screening mammography, routine quality metric assessment set forth by the steering committee is necessary to address potential opportunities or deficiencies in a timely manner. The quality indicators presented in 3.2.2 are examples of program quality indicators [69]. The following list of metrics is another example of metrics that the steering committee could follow on an annual or quarterly basis, Table 3.6 [76]:

Table 3.6 Quality metrics and care escalation

ACCESS	• Number Referred[1] • Number Qualified • Number Scanned • Number Enrolled • Number Discharged • Referral Source
SMOKING	• Number Current • Number Former • Number Quit[1] • Number Relapsed[1]
RADIOLOGY	• Lung-RADSTM Category[3] • S Positive[3] • Coronary Calcs[3] • Emphysema[3]
CANCER DETECTION RATE	• Stage • Histology • Presumed[4]
NON-INVASIVE PROCEDURES	• Pulmonary Consults • PET/CT
INVASIVE PROCEDURES	• Percutaneous Biopsy • Bronch w/Biopsy • Surgery • Benign Disease

[1]Overall and by provider
[2]How heard about program
[3]Overall and by radiologist
[4]PET positive, growth and multidisciplinary consensus

3.3.6 Research Oversight

Clinical research is necessary for future advances in LCS. Steering committees associated with academic centers should interface with a dedicated research committee to ratify clinical research initiatives and industry research partnerships.

3.4 Navigation

Teresa Giamboy

3.4.1 Introduction

Navigating patients through any health journey is a comprehensive process that may include a variety of different approaches in order to care for patients. These diverse models offer expertise and guidance from different stakeholders, perhaps in different departments, or even different organizations, but have the common goal of coordinating care for patients and seeing them through the health care continuum. Patient navigators assist patients in accessing care and guide them through the health care system, helping them overcome identified individual barriers [77]. A variety of barriers may effect a patient's desire to seek preventative care, and navigation has proven to be a successful tool to combat disparities among vulnerable populations [78]. In the case of lung cancer screening (LCS), navigation can be applied in many unique ways, as the patient will travel through numerous pathways to complete the preventative care process, all of which host an opportunity to navigate the patient. The goal of navigation is to decrease burden to the patient and assist in timely care delivery through coordination and increased communication [79]. Navigation helps to connect the dots for the patient, which increases adherence to care, as they are directly supported throughout the process.

3.4.2 Office/Department-Based Navigation

Once a patient is identified as meeting the eligibility for lung cancer screening, as determined through a shared decision-making discussion with a provider, they will be directed to obtain a lung cancer screening CT scan. If there is a patient navigator in the office of the referring provider, that navigator can serve as the facilitator for the process. The tasks of the navigator may include assisting in insurance authorizations, scheduling the low-dose CT scan and communicating that to the patient, completing any necessary forms required by radiology, and ensuring the results reach the ordering provider for prompt review.

The challenge with this level of navigation in a primary care or a specialist office is the large volume of patients and countless needs for each patient. This has not been a model frequently implemented given the complexity of polymorbidity in the general patient population, the dynamic patient care that occurs in these practices [80], and the large volume of tasks that are shunted to the patient. Research shows that patients recall a minority of what their provider discussed with them after leaving the office [81], which further derails recommended care.

Department-based navigation also offers additional challenges, as the ordering provider and performing facility may utilize different electronic medical records (EMR), which do not interface with each other. EMRs have incredible potential in functionality focused on disease surveillance and prevention capabilities; however, availability of a sophisticated platform is required for accuracy and comprehensiveness [82]. The possibility of not receiving lung cancer screening results could delay the care of a possible malignancy, or concerning incidental finding, particularly if a prompt response or intervention is recommended. Having designated navigation teams focused on the screening process and outcomes could help to facilitate increased communication between departments.

3.4.3 Lung Cancer Screening Program Navigation

The lung cancer screening specific navigation model has become the preferred model by patients and healthcare teams alike, as it removes the burden of coordinating the process while allowing dedicated clinical personnel to assist in managing and tracking participants and program quality. Centralized screening programs with navigation emerged as the independent factor most strongly associated with annual adherence to screening [83]. The tasks managed by a program navigator may include determining eligibility and risk stratification, appropriate documentation and ordering, tobacco counseling and treatment planning, authorizing, scheduling, and communicating appointments to participants, reviewing results with the multidisciplinary team and reviewing recommendations with patients, assisting in data management and regulatory requirements, assisting patients in additional care needs based on the findings, and coordinating higher levels of care to additional interdisciplinary team members when appropriate. Communicating with program participants throughout each step of the process is key to their engagement and continued adherence, particularly when abnormal findings are detected and warrant additional diagnostic evaluation.

3.4.4   The Benefit of Nursing Navigation in Cancer Screening

The benefit to navigating screening participants is obvious; coordinating care increases the likelihood that participants make it through each step in the process. However, there is an even greater benefit in having a nurse serve as the navigator. Nurses have a strong educational background in health care and can field more complex questions and concerns from participants, while also having the bandwidth to communicate effectively with the interdisciplinary care teams. Nurse navigators provide instrumental and emotional support, address barriers to patient care, coordinate referrals, and strengthen patient–provider relationships [84]. This work helps to support more robust screening program rates, adherence to annual and follow-up screening, shortening time to treatment, increased patient satisfaction, and improved quality of life for the patient [78].

3.4.5   Navigating Lung Cancer Screening in the Electronic Medical Record

The complexity of lung cancer screening navigation creates challenges to effective navigation, which has prompted many organizations to turn to their electronic medical record (EMR) and/or a third party software system for automated support. With a variety of vendors and programs on the market, each institution needs to determine what would work best for them. Variables to consider include cost, quality, interface-capability with the EMR, and overall effectiveness. The end-user is often the best party to trial these programs, while the administrative team ultimately determines what is feasible for the organization financially.

An interfaced software or EMR-driven model would be the ideal solution, so that information can be found and managed in one system directly linked to the patient's medical record. EMR capability to accurately calculate pack-years and identify eligible participants for lung cancer screening remains an enigma for most, as functionality. Even the most advanced and established centralized lung screening programs find this to be a significant barrier to uptake of screening. The integration of LCS-specific software with existing EMRs is increasingly crucial for organizations to be able to deliver evidence-based, compliant care that is properly reimbursed [85].

EMR-based management and tracking becomes even more important when overseeing incidental findings on lung cancer screening scans. By working within one system, reviewing of historic imaging and documentation is helpful for radiology, and a centralized screening program alike, to determine if there is a need for additional testing, follow-up, or intervention.

Navigators play a key role in this facet of care, as they are often the communicators between the patient and their care team, very importantly the primary care provider and related specialists. If an abnormal incidental finding is detected, and perhaps requires rapid evaluation by another specialist, navigators can work with their colleagues to elevate this case for fast-track review and evaluation, which could be lifesaving to a patient.

3.4.6 Navigation Summary

The benefit of navigation in the lung cancer screening realm benefits patients through coordinated care delivery, result/recommendation facilitation and management, and fast-tracking necessary care when appropriate. This model offers incredible advantages to program participants, particularly if abnormal findings are detected and require additional intervention, but also for the large majority of patients who are found to have non-suspicious lung screening scans and simply require annual follow-up. Navigation increases adherence to ongoing preventative care and serves as the central point of contact for participants during all legs of their journey [86].

References

1. Fontana RS, Sanderson DR, Woolner LB, Taylor WF, Miller WE, Muhm JR. Lung cancer screening: the Mayo program. J Occup Environ Med. 1986;28(8):746–50.
2. Brett GZ. The value of lung cancer detection by six-monthly chest radiographs. Thorax. 1968;23(4):414–20.
3. Melamed MR, Flehinger BJ, Zaman MB, Heelan RT, Perchick WA, Martini N. Screening for early lung cancer. Results of the Memorial Sloan-Kettering study in New York. Chest. 1984;86(1):44–53.
4. Brawley OW. Cancer screening. Cancer Prev Screen. 2018:31–40.
5. McCaffery KJ, Jacklyn GL, Barratt A, Brodersen J, Glasziou P, Carter SM, Hicks NR, Howard K, Irwig L. Recommendations about screening. In: Guyatt G, Rennie D, Meade MO, Cook DJ, editors. Users' guides to the medical literature: a manual for evidence-based clinical practice. 3rd ed. New York: McGraw-Hill Education; 2015.
6. Tockman MS. Survival and mortality from lung cancer in a screened population: the Johns Hopkins Study. Chest. 1986;89(4 Suppl):324S–5S.
7. Marcus PM, Bergstralh EJ, Fagerstrom RM, Williams DE, Fontana R, Taylor WF, Prorok PC. Lung cancer mortality in the Mayo Lung Project: impact of extended follow-up. J Natl Cancer Inst. 2000;92(16):1308–16.
8. Oken MM, Hocking WG, Kvale PA, Andriole GL, Buys SS, Church TR, Crawford ED, Fouad MN, Isaacs C, Reding DJ, Weissfeld JL, Yokochi LA, O'Brien B, Ragard LR, Rathmell JM, Riley TL, Wright P, Caparaso N, Hu P, et al. Screening by chest radiograph and lung cancer mortality: the prostate, lung, colorectal, and ovarian (PLCO) randomized trial. JAMA. 2011;306(17):1865–73.
9. Sone S, Nakayama T, Honda T, Tsushima K, Li F, Haniuda M, Takahashi Y, Suzuki T, Yamanda T, Kondo R, Hanaoka T, Takayama F, Kubo K, Fushimi H. Long-term follow-up study of a

population-based 1996-1998 mass screening programme for lung cancer using mobile low-dose spiral computed tomography. Lung Cancer. 2007;58(3):329–41.

10. Henschke CI, McCauley DI, Yankelevitz DF, Naidich DP, McGuinness G, Miettinen OS, Libby DM, Pasmantier MW, Koizumi J, Altorki NK, Smith JP. Early Lung Cancer Action Project: overall design and findings from baseline screening. Lancet. 1999;354(9173):99–105.

11. International Early Lung Cancer Action Program Investigators, Henschke CI, Yankelevitz DF, Libby DM, Pasmantier MW, Smith JP, Miettinen OS. Survival of patients with stage I lung cancer detected on CT screening. N Engl J Med. 2006;355(17):1763–71.

12. Howlader N, Noone AM, Krapcho M, Miller D, Bishop K, Altekruse SF, Kosary CL, Yu M, Ruhl J, Tatalovich Z, Mariotto A, Lewis DR, Chen HS, Feuer EJCK, editors. SEER cancer statistics review, 1975–2013. Bethesda: National Cancer Institute; 2015.

13. Sobue T, Moriyama N, Kaneko M, Kusumoto M, Kobayashi T, Tsuchiya R, Kakinuma R, Ohmatsu H, Nagai K, Nishiyama H, Matsui E, Eguchi K. Screening for lung cancer with low-dose helical computed tomography: anti-lung cancer association project. J Clin Oncol. 2002;20(4):911–20.

14. Team NLSTR, Aberle DR, Adams AM, Berg CD, Black WC, Clapp JD, Fagerstrom RM, Gareen IF, Gatsonis C, Marcus PM, Sicks JD. Reduced lung-cancer mortality with low-dose computed tomographic screening. N Engl J Med. 2011;365(5):395–409.

15. National Lung Screening Trial Research Team. Lung cancer incidence and mortality with extended follow-up in the National Lung Screening Trial. J Thorac Oncol. 2019;14(10):1732–42.

16. Tanner NT, Gebregziabher M, Hughes Halbert C, Payne E, Egede LE, Silvestri GA. Racial differences in outcomes within the National Lung Screening Trial. Implications for widespread implementation. Am J Respir Crit Care Med. 2015;192(2):200–8.

17. Goulart BHL, Ramsey SD. Moving beyond the National Lung Screening Trial: discussing strategies for implementation of Lung Cancer Screening Programs. Oncologist. 2013;18(8):941–6.

18. Aberle DR, Adams AM, Berg CD, Clapp JD, Clingan KL, Gareen IF, Lynch DA, Marcus PM, Pinsky PF. Baseline characteristics of participants in the randomized National Lung Screening Trial. J Natl Cancer Inst. 2010;102(23):1771–9.

19. Field JK, van Klaveren R, Pedersen JH, Pastorino U, Paci E, Becker N, Infante M, Oudkerk M, de Koning HJ. European randomized lung cancer screening trials: post NLST. J Surg Oncol. 2013;108(5):280–6.

20. Oudkerk M, Devaraj A, Vliegenthart R, Henzler T, Prosch H, Heussel CP, Bastarrika G, Sverzellati N, Mascalchi M, Delorme S, Baldwin DR, Callister ME, Becker N, Heuvelmans MA, Rzyman W, Infante MV, Pastorino U, Pedersen JH, Paci E, et al. European position statement on lung cancer screening. Lancet Oncol. 2017;18(12):e754–66.

21. van Klaveren RJ, Oudkerk M, Prokop M, Scholten ET, Nackaerts K, Vernhout R, van Iersel CA, van den Bergh KAM, van't Westeinde S, van der Aalst C, Thunnissen E, Xu DM, Wang Y, Zhao Y, Gietema HA, de Hoop BJ, Groen HJM, de Bock GH, van Ooijen P, et al. Management of lung nodules detected by volume CT scanning. N Engl J Med. 2009;361(23):2221–9.

22. Wille MMW, Dirksen A, Ashraf H, Saghir Z, Bach KS, Brodersen J, Clementsen PF, Hansen H, Larsen KR, Mortensen J, Rasmussen JF, Seersholm N, Skov BG, Thomsen LH, Tønnesen P, Pedersen JH. Results of the randomized Danish Lung Cancer Screening Trial with focus on high-risk profiling. Am J Respir Crit Care Med. 2016;193(5):542–51.

23. Becker N, Motsch E, Gross ML, Eigentopf A, Heussel CP, Dienemann H, Schnabel PA, Eichinger M, Optazaite DE, Puderbach M, Wielpütz M, Kauczor HU, Tremper J, Delorme S. Randomized study on early detection of lung cancer with MSCT in Germany: results of the first 3 years of follow-up after randomization. J Thorac Oncol. 2015;10(6):890–6.

24. Field JK, Duffy SW, Baldwin DR, Brain KE, Devaraj A, Eisen T, Green BA, Holemans JA, Kavanagh T, Kerr KM, Ledson M, Lifford KJ, McRonald FE, Nair A, Page RD, Parmar MK, Rintoul RC, Screaton N, Wald NJ, et al. The UK Lung Cancer Screening Trial: a pilot randomised controlled trial of low-dose computed tomography screening for the early detection of lung cancer. Health Technol Assess. 2016;20(40):1–146.

25. Berg CD, Fong KM, Marshall HM. Lung cancer screening. Cancer Prev Screen. 2018;28:237–55.

26. Silva M, Pastorino U, Sverzellati N. Lung cancer screening with low-dose CT in Europe: strength and weakness of diverse independent screening trials. Clin Radiol. 2017;72(5):389–400.

27. van Iersel CA, de Koning HJ, Draisma G, Mali WPTM, Scholten ET, Nackaerts K, Prokop M, Habbema JDF, Oudkerk M, van Klaveren RJ. Risk-based selection from the general population in a screening trial: selection criteria, recruitment and power for the Dutch-Belgian randomised lung cancer multi-slice CT screening trial (NELSON). Int J Cancer. 2007;120(4):868–74.

28. de Koning HJ, van der Aalst CM, de Jong PA, Scholten ET, Nackaerts K, Heuvelmans MA, Lammers JWJ, Weenink C, Yousaf-Khan U, Horeweg N, van't Westeinde S, Prokop M, Mali WP, Mohamed Hoesein FAA, van Ooijen PMA, Aerts JGJV, den Bakker MA, Thunnissen E, Verschakelen J, et al. Reduced lung-cancer mortality with volume CT screening in a randomized trial. N Engl J Med. 2020;382(6):503–13.

29. Patz EFJ, Pinsky P, Gatsonis C, Sicks JD, Kramer BS, Tammemägi MC, Chiles C, Black WC, Aberle DR. Overdiagnosis in low-dose computed tomography screening for lung cancer. JAMA Intern Med. 2014;174(2):269–74.

30. Pinsky PF, Berg CD. Applying the National Lung Screening Trial eligibility criteria to the US population: what percent of the population and of incident lung cancers would be covered? J Med Screen. 2012;19(3):154–6.

31. Meza R, Jeon J, Toumazis I, ten Haaf K, Cao P, Bastani M, Han SS, Blom EF, Jonas DE, Feuer EJ, Plevritis SK, de Koning HJ, Kong CY. Evaluation of the benefits and harms of lung cancer screening with low-dose computed tomography: modeling study for the US Preventive Services Task Force. JAMA. 2021;325(10):988–97.

32. Force USPST. Screening for lung cancer: US Preventive Services Task Force recommendation statement. JAMA. 2021;325(10):962–70.

33. Draft evidence review: lung cancer: screening | United States Preventive Services Taskforce.

34. Jonas DE, Reuland DS, Reddy SM, Nagle M, Clark SD, Weber RP, Enyioha C, Malo TL, Brenner AT, Armstrong C, Coker-Schwimmer M, Middleton JC, Voisin C, Harris RP. Screening for lung cancer with low-dose computed tomography: updated evidence report and systematic review for the US Preventive Services Task Force. JAMA. 2021;325(10):971–87.

35. Moyer VA, Force USPST. Screening for lung cancer: U.S. Preventive Services Task Force recommendation statement. Ann Intern Med. 2014;160(5):330–4.

36. Rivera MP, Tanner NT, Silvestri GA, Detterbeck FC, Tammemägi MC, Young RP, Slatore CG, Caverly TJ, Boyd CM, Braithwaite D, Fathi JT, Gould MK, Iaccarino JM, Malkoski SP, Mazzone PJ, Tanoue LT, Schoenborn NL, Zulueta JJ, Wiener RS. Incorporating coexisting chronic illness into decisions about patient selection for lung cancer screening. An Official American Thoracic Society Research Statement. Am J Respir Crit Care Med. 2018;198(2):e3–13.

37. Katki HA, Kovalchik SA, Petito LC, Cheung LC, Jacobs E, Jemal A, Berg CD, Chaturvedi AK. Implications of nine risk prediction models for selecting ever-smokers for computed tomography lung cancer screening. Ann Intern Med. 2018;169(1):10–9.

38. Kauczor HU, Baird AM, Blum TG, Bonomo L, Bostantzoglou C, Burghuber O, Čepická B, Comanescu A, Couraud S, Devaraj A, Jespersen V, Morozov S, Nardi Agmon I, Peled N, Powell P, Prosch H, Ravara S, Rawlinson J, Revel MP, et al. ESR/ERS statement paper on lung cancer screening. Eur Respir J. 2020;55(2):1900506.

39. Mazzone PJ, Silvestri GA, Souter LH, Caverly TJ, Kanne JP, Katki HA, Wiener RS, Detterbeck FC. Screening for lung cancer: CHEST guideline and expert panel report. Chest. 2021;160(5):e427–94.

40. Brenner DJ. Radiation risks potentially associated with low-dose CT screening of adult smokers for lung cancer. Radiology. 2004;231(2):440–5.

41. Davies L, Petitti DB, Martin L, Woo M, Lin JS. Defining, estimating, and communicating overdiagnosis in cancer screening. Ann Intern Med. 2018;169(1):36–43.

42. Brodersen J, Voss T, Martiny F, Siersma V, Barratt A, Heleno B. Overdiagnosis of lung cancer with low-dose computed tomography screening: meta-analysis of the randomised clinical trials. Breathe. 2020;16(1):200013.

43. Pinsky PF. Assessing the benefits and harms of low-dose computed tomography screening for lung cancer. Lung Cancer Manag. 2014;3(6):491–8.

44. Pinsky PF, Gierada DS, Black W, Munden R, Nath H, Aberle D, Kazerooni E. Performance of lung-RADS in the National Lung Screening Trial: a retrospective assessment. Ann Intern Med. 2015;162(7):485–91.

45. Wu GX, Raz DJ, Brown L, Sun V. Psychological burden associated with lung cancer screening: a systematic review. Clin Lung Cancer. 2016;17(5):315–24.

46. Smetana GW, Boiselle PM, Schwartzstein RM. Screening for lung cancer with low-dose computed tomography. Ann Intern Med. 2015;162(8):577–82.

47. Centers for Medicare & Medicaid. Decision memo for screening for lung cancer with low dose computed tomography (LDCT) (CAG-00439N).

48. Nishi SPE, Lowenstein LM, Mendoza TR, Lopez Olivo MA, Crocker LC, Sepucha K, Niu J, Volk RJ. Shared decision-making for lung cancer screening: how well are we "sharing"? Chest. 2021;160(1):330–40.

49. Mazzone PJ, Tenenbaum A, Seeley M, Petersen H, Lyon C, Han X, Wang XF. Impact of a lung cancer screening counseling and shared decision-making visit. Chest. 2017;151(3):572–8.

50. Hoffmann TC, Del Mar C. Clinicians' expectations of the benefits and harms of treatments, screening, and tests: a systematic review. JAMA Intern Med. 2017;177(3):407–19.

51. Hoffmann TC, Del Mar C. Patients' expectations of the benefits and harms of treatments, screening, and tests: a systematic review. JAMA Intern Med. 2015;175(2):274–86.

52. Toumazis I, de Nijs K, Cao P, Bastani M, Munshi V, ten Haaf K, Jeon J, Gazelle GS, Feuer EJ, de Koning HJ, Meza R, Kong CY, Han SS, Plevritis SK. Cost-effectiveness evaluation of the 2021 US Preventive Services Task Force recommendation for lung cancer screening. JAMA Oncol. 2021;7(12):1833–42.

53. Lococo F, Cardillo G, Veronesi G. Does a lung cancer screening programme promote smoking cessation? Thorax. 2017;72(10):870–1.

54. Filippo L, Principe R, Cesario A, Apolone G, Carleo F, Ialongo P, Veronesi G, Cardillo G. Smoking cessation intervention within the framework of a lung cancer screening program: preliminary results and clinical perspectives from the "Cosmos-II" trial. Lung. 2015;193(1):147–9.

55. Deppen SA, Grogan EL, Aldrich MC, Massion PP. Lung cancer screening and smoking cessation: a teachable moment? J Natl Cancer Inst. 2014;106(6):dju122.

56. van der Aalst CM, van den Bergh KAM, Willemsen MC, de Koning HJ, van Klaveren RJ. Lung cancer screening and smoking abstinence: 2 year follow-up data from the Dutch–Belgian randomised controlled lung cancer screening trial. Thorax. 2010;65(7):600–5.

57. Ashraf H, Tønnesen P, Holst Pedersen J, Dirksen A, Thorsen H, Døssing M. Effect of CT screening on smoking habits at 1-year follow-up in the Danish Lung Cancer Screening Trial (DLCST). Thorax. 2009;64(5):388–92.

58. Clark MA, Gorelick JJ, Sicks JD, Park ER, Graham AL, Abrams DB, Gareen IF. The relations between false positive and negative screens and smoking cessation and relapse in the National Lung Screening Trial: implications for public health. Nicotine Tob Res. 2015;18(1):17–24.

59. Morgan L, Choi H, Reid M, Khawaja A, Mazzone PJ. Frequency of incidental findings and subsequent evaluation in low-dose computed tomographic scans for lung cancer screening. Ann Am Thorac Soc. 2017;14(9):1450–6.

60. Mendoza DP, Kako B, Digumarthy SR, Shepard JAO, Little BP. Impact of significant coronary artery calcification reported on low-dose computed tomography lung cancer screening. J Thorac Imaging. 2020;35(2):129–35.

61. Munden RF, Carter BW, Chiles C, MacMahon H, Black WC, Ko JP, McAdams HP, Rossi SE, Leung AN, Boiselle PM, Kent MS, Brown K, Dyer DS, Hartman TE, Goodman EM, Naidich DP, Kazerooni EA, Berland LL, Pandharipande PV. Managing incidental findings on thoracic

CT: mediastinal and cardiovascular findings. A White Paper of the ACR Incidental Findings Committee. J Am Coll Radiol. 2018;15(8):1087–96.

62. Tammemägi MC, Church TR, Hocking WG, Silvestri GA, Kvale PA, Riley TL, Commins J, Berg CD. Evaluation of the lung cancer risks at which to screen ever- and never-smokers: screening rules applied to the PLCO and NLST cohorts. PLoS Med. 2014;11(12):e1001764.

63. Ardila D, Kiraly AP, Bharadwaj S, Choi B, Reicher JJ, Peng L, Tse D, Etemadi M, Ye W, Corrado G, Naidich DP, Shetty S. End-to-end lung cancer screening with three-dimensional deep learning on low-dose chest computed tomography. Nat Med. 2019;25(6):954–61.

64. Choi HK, Wang X, Mazzone PJ. Artificial intelligence as a diagnostic tool for lung nodule evaluation. J Med Artif Intell Online First. Published online; 2020.

65. Cherezov D, Hawkins SH, Goldgof DB, Hall LO, Liu Y, Li Q, Balagurunathan Y, Gillies RJ, Schabath MB. Delta radiomic features improve prediction for lung cancer incidence: a nested case-control analysis of the National Lung Screening Trial. Cancer Med. 2018;7(12):6340–56.

66. Fujita M, Higaki T, Awaya Y, Nakanishi T, Nakamura Y, Tatsugami F, Baba Y, Iida M, Awai K. Lung cancer screening with ultra-low dose CT using full iterative reconstruction. Jpn J Radiol. 2017;35(4):179–89.

67. HEDIS-NCQA. Published 2021. Accessed 26 Jan 2022. https://www.ncqa.org/hedis/.

68. National Academies of Science E and M. Implementation of lung cancer screening: proceedings of a workshop; 2017.

69. Mazzone PJ, White CS, Kazerooni EA, Smith RA, Thomson CC. Proposed quality metrics for lung cancer screening programs: a National Lung Cancer Roundtable Project. Chest. 2021;160(1):368–78. https://doi.org/10.1016/j.chest.2021.01.063.

70. National Center for Health Statistics. Survey description, National Health Interview Survey; 2015. www.cdc.gov/nchs/nhis/data-questionnaires-documentation.htm.

71. Office of Disease Prevention and Health Promotion. Increase the proportion of adults who get screened for lung cancer—C-03—healthy people 2030 | health.gov. Published 2021. Accessed 26 Jan 2022. https://health.gov/healthypeople/objectives-and-data/browse-objectives/cancer/increase-proportion-adults-who-get-screened-lung-cancer-c-03.

72. American Thoracic Society/American Lung Association Lung Cancer Screening Implementation Guide: https://www.lungcancerscreeningguide.org/initiating-a-lung-cancer-screening-program/program-structure/.

73. McKee AB, McKee BJ, Wald C, et al. Rescue lung, rescue life: translating the national lung screening trial results into clinical practice. Oncol Issues. 2014;29(2):20–9.

74. McKee BJ, McKee AB, Flacke S, et al. Initial experience with a free, high-volume, low-dose CT lung cancer screening program. J Am Coll Radiol. 2013;10(8):586–92.

75. Price EL, Bereknyei S, Kuby A, et al. New elements for informed decision making: a qualitative study of older adults' views. Patient Educ Couns. 2012;86(3):335–41.

76. American Thoracic Society/American Lung Association Lung Cancer Screening Implementation Guide. https://www.lungcancerscreeningguide.org/program-navigation-and-data-tracking/planning-an-lcs-program/.

77. Percac-Lima S, Ashburner JM, Zai AH, et al. Patient navigation for comprehensive cancer screening in high-risk patients using a population-based health information technology system: a randomized clinical trial. JAMA Intern Med. 2016;176(7):930–7. https://doi.org/10.1001/jamainternmed.2016.0841.

78. Shusted CS, Barta JA, Lake M, Brawer R, Ruane B, Giamboy TE, Sundaram B, Evans NR, Myers RE, Kane GC. The case for patient navigation in lung cancer screening in vulnerable populations: a systematic review. Popul Health Manag. 2019;22(4):347–61. https://doi.org/10.1089/pop.2018.0128. Epub 2018 Nov 8. PMID: 30407102; PMCID: PMC6685525.

79. Freeman H. The origin, evolution, and principles of patient navigation. Cancer Epidemiol Biomarkers Prev. 2012;21(10):1614–7. https://doi.org/10.1158/1055-9965.EPI-12-0982.

80. Carter N, et al. Navigation delivery models and roles of navigators in primary care: a scoping literature review. BMC Health Serv Res. 2018;18(1):96. https://doi.org/10.1186/s12913-018-2889-0.

81. Cleveland Clinic. Why we forget what the doctor told us (and what to do about it). 2019. https://health.clevelandclinic.org/why-we-forget-what-the-doctor-told-us-and-what-to-do-about-it/.

82. Kruse CS, Stein A, Thomas H, Kaur H. The use of electronic health records to support population health: a systematic review of the literature. J Med Syst. 2018;42(11):214. https://doi.org/10.1007/s10916-018-1075-6. PMID: 30269237; PMCID: PMC6182727.

83. Sakoda LC, et al. Patterns and factors associated with adherence to lung cancer screening in diverse practice settings. JAMA Netw Open. 2021;4(4):e218559. https://doi.org/10.1001/jamanetworkopen.2021.8559.

84. Gerber D, Gillam A, Hamann H. Lung cancer screening in the "real world" and the role of nurse navigators. J Oncol Navig Surviv. 2013;4(2). https://www.jons-online.com/issues/2013/april-2013-vol-4-no-2/1229-lung-cancer-screening-in-the-real-world-and-the-role-of-nurse-navigators#:~:text=How%20Can%20Nurse%20Navigation%20Be,and%20strengthen%20patient%2Dprovider%20relationships.

85. Fathi JT, White CS, Greenberg GM, Mazzone PJ, Smith RA, Thomson CC. The integral role of the electronic health record and tracking software in the implementation of lung cancer screening—a call to action to developers: a White Paper from the National Lung Cancer Roundtable. Chest. 2020;157(6):1674–9. https://doi.org/10.1016/j.chest.2019.12.004. Epub 2019 Dec 23. PMID: 31877270.

86. Kelly R. Defining the role of the oncology nurse and patient navigator. Cranbury: Academy of Oncology Nurse & Patient Navigators; 2021. https://aonnonline.org/expert-commentary/aonn-blog/3609-defining-the-role-of-the-oncology-nurse-and-patient-navigator

Chapter 4
Implementing Lung Cancer Screening in Clinical Practice

Janelle V. Baptiste, Julie Barta, Sahil Patel, Carey C. Thomson, Melissa Tukey, and Gaetane Michaud

J. V. Baptiste (✉)
Division of Pulmonary, Critical Care & Sleep Medicine, Beth Israel Deaconess Medical Center, Harvard Medical School, Boston, MA, USA
e-mail: jbaptis4@bidmc.harvard.edu

J. Barta
Jane and Leonard Korman Respiratory Institute, Division of Pulmonary and Critical Care Medicine, Thomas Jefferson University, Philadelphia, PA, USA

S. Patel
Pulmonary, Critical Care, Sleep Medicine, Massachusetts General Hospital/Beth Israel Deaconess Medical Center Combined Fellowship Program, Boston, MA, USA

C. C. Thomson
Mt Auburn Hospital, Harvard Medical School, Cambridge, MA, USA

M. Tukey
Medicine, Interventional Pulmonology, University of South Florida Morsani College of Medicine, Tampa, FL, USA

G. Michaud
Medicine and Cardiothoracic Surgery, Pulmonary, Critical Care and Sleep Medicine, University of South Florida Morsani College of Medicine, Tampa, FL, USA

© The Author(s), under exclusive license to Springer Nature
Switzerland AG 2022
J. V. Baptiste et al. (eds.), *Lung Cancer Screening*,
https://doi.org/10.1007/978-3-031-10662-0_4

57

4.1   Lung Cancer Screening Eligibility Criteria and Confirmation of Eligibility

4.1.1   Current Eligibility Criteria for Lung Cancer Screening

Lung cancer screening (LCS) with low-dose computed tomography (LDCT) is a complex, multistep process that involves assessing an individual's eligibility for screening, shared decision making, acquiring and interpreting images, communication and management of imaging findings. Determining an individual's eligibility for screening is an important first step in the process of LDCT screening. Trials investigating LDCT screening have predominantly focused on selecting individuals based on minimum and maximum age limits plus summary indices of cumulative lifetime smoking exposure [1]. These inclusion criteria inherently represent a form of risk-based selection of participants but are motivated by statistical power considerations that aim to obtain a sufficiently high average lung cancer risk for the study population as a whole, rather than on individual risk [2, 3].

Although most of the clinical practice guidelines have eligibility criteria that are consistent with the NLST in terms of pack-year smoking history, and age, a few have since gone on to expand their eligibility criteria beyond that of the NLST [Table 4.1]. Studies investigating limitations to using NLST eligibility criteria only report on oversimplification of risk for lung cancer, ignoring well-known risk factors, and screening of persons at lower risk of lung cancer as strong evidence for expanding screening guidelines in clinical practice [4–6]. The United States Preventive Services Task Force (USPSTF), the National Comprehensive Cancer Network (NCCN), and the Centers for Medicare and Medicaid Services (CMS) are three organizations which have expanded their screening eligibility guidelines beyond that of the NLST criteria. In 2014, the USPSTF used modeling to determine the optimum screening policy for lung cancer screening in a US cohort born in 1950, and followed from ages 45 to 90 years. This led to a change in the eligibility requirements for lung cancer screening to include screening eligibility up to age 80 years, expanding beyond the 74 year cut-off in NLST [7]. The National Comprehensive Cancer Network (NCCN) also extrapolated from other studies and models to expand their eligibility criteria to include an additional risk factor for lung cancer. In the pooled analysis from Brenner et al., lung cancer risk was found to be 2.44 times higher in those with emphysema [8]. In addition, McKee et al. comparing results from high-risk individuals meeting NLST criteria with the expanded high-risk group identified by the NCCN criteria (ages 50–55 with 20 pack-year smoking history and an additional risk factor) were able to show that the expanded risk category was substantially similar to the NLST group in terms of positive screening results and lung cancer diagnoses; suggesting extra lives saved each year with expanding screening eligibility to include this high-risk group [9]. CMS which provides national coverage determination for a number of individuals over the age of 74, and more likely to be diagnosed with lung cancer, took the approach of convening the Medicare Evidence Development and Coverage Advisory Committee (MEDCAC) to review the evidence and provide guidance on screening eligibility criteria [10]. After convening several meetings with MEDCAC, national coverage of LDCT screening was recommended for

Table 4.1 Overview of the current eligibility criteria for LDCT lung cancer screening

Organizations	Eligibility criteria
U.S. Preventive Services Task Force (USPSTF)	The USPSTF recommends annual screening for lung cancer with low-dose computed tomography in adults ages 50–80 years who have a 20 pack-year smoking history and currently smoke or have quit within the past 15 years. Screening should be discontinued once a person has not smoked for 15 years or develops a health problem that substantially limits life expectancy or the ability or willingness to have curative lung surgery.
Centers for Medicare and Medicaid Services National Coverage Determination on Lung Cancer Screening (CMS)	People ages 55–77 with at least a 30 pack-year smoking history and who currently smoke or have quit within the past 15 years.
	Medicare coverage includes a visit for counseling and shared decision making on the potential benefits and risks of lung cancer screening. The National Coverage Determination also includes required data collection and specific coverage eligibility criteria for radiologists and radiology imaging centers, consistent with the National Lung Screening Trial (NLST) protocol, USPSTF recommendation, and multisociety, multidisciplinary, stakeholder evidence-based guidelines.
Clinical Practice Guidelines from ACCP, ACS, ALA, ASCO, ATS, IASLC	Follow the NLST eligibility criteria. People ages 55, with variability in stopping age by organization with at least a 30 pack-year smoking history and who currently or formerly smoke.
National Comprehensive Cancer Network (NCCN)	People ages 55–74 with at least a 30 pack-year smoking history and who currently smoke or have quit within 15 years. People ages 50 and older with at least a 20 pack-year smoking history and an additional risk factor for lung cancer. Additional risk factors include occupational or environmental exposures, a personal or family history of cancer, and additional lung disease such as COPD and pulmonary fibrosis, but not second-hand smoking. The same criteria are recommended by the American Academy of thoracic surgeons.
American Academy of Family Physicians (AAFP)	The evidence is sufficient evidence to support a B recommendation for LCS in adults. Supports the USPSTF 2021 recommendation for LCS in adults ages 50–80 years who have a 20 pack-year smoking history and currently smoke or have quit within the past 15 years. Screening should be discontinued once a person has not smoked for 15 years or develops a health problem that substantially limits life expectancy or the ability or willingness to have curative lung surgery.

NOTE: *ACCP* American College of Chest Physicians, *ACS* American Cancer Society, *ALA* American Lung Association, *ASCO* American Society of Clinical Oncology, *ATS* American Thoracic Society, *IASLC* International Association for the Study of Lung Cancer, *LDCT* low-dose computed tomography. SOURCES: Adapted from Bach, Chin, LeFevre, and Wood presentations, June 20, 2016; Borgmeyer, 2014; CMS, 2015; Wood et al., 2012. Adapted from: National Academic of Sciences, Engineering, and Medicine, 2017. Implementation of Lung Cancer Screening: Proceedings of a workshop. https://doi.org/10.17226/23680. Reproduced with permission from the National Academy of Sciences, Courtesy of the National Academies Press, Washington, DC

Medicare beneficiaries up to age 77 years, who are asymptomatic and have at least a 30 pack-year smoking history and are current smokers or have quit smoking within the past 15 years [10]. In addition, CMS also mandates a number of requirements for coverage. These requirements include: clinicians' determination of an individual's eligibility for screening and understanding of benefits and risk of screening; individual's participation in tobacco cessation counseling and a shared decision-making visit prior to LDCT screening; and criteria that radiologists must meet for LDCT screening [10]. In this section, we will focus on meeting the requirement of determining and ensuring eligibility of an individual for lung cancer screening (LCS).

4.1.2   Determining and Ensuring Eligibility for Lung Cancer Screening (LCS)

Determining eligibility for LCS with LDCT can occur at the individual level or at the program level. At the individual level, primary care providers (PCPs) are often the first point of contact for an individual during the screening process. PCPs are responsible for talking with individuals about LDCT screening and assessing their eligibility for LDCT screening. PCPs also provide referrals for follow-up and orders for further LDCT screening scans. As a result, PCPs need to be fully knowledgeable of the eligibility requirements which an individual must meet for LDCT screening. However, in surveys conducted in 4 US states from 2013 and 2015, between 49% and 86% of survey respondents were aware of LCS guidelines [11–13]. More specifically, there was a low awareness of how frequently screening should occur and the age at which screening should conclude. Some study respondents also expressed concern over potential changes that could be made to the USPSTF recommendations on length of screening or who to screen because of new evidence. Raz and colleagues, in their survey of PCPs also showed that less than half of surveyed PCPs were aware of USPSTF recommendations on the use of LDCT scans for LCS, and only 12% of the surveyed PCPs referred their eligible patients for screening [14]. In 2021, the 2013 USPSTF recommendation statement on LCS with LDCT was updated to include initiation of screening at the lower age of 50 years and a lesser pack-year smoking history based on new evidence [15]. To date, there are no published studies assessing PCPs' knowledge and awareness of the 2021 USPSTF recommendations.

The first step in determining an individual's eligibility for LCS is ensuring that the individual is asymptomatic at the time of screening. All recommendations for LDCT screening specify that an individual should be asymptomatic at the time of screening [Table 4.1]. Individuals with signs and symptoms that could be consistent with lung cancer such as hemoptysis (coughing up of blood), unexplained weight loss, and night sweats are ineligible for screening with LDCT and instead should undergo a diagnostic chest computed tomography scan. However, determining whether an individual who smokes is asymptomatic or not, and still eligible for LCS is often more challenging. Current and former smokers can report a longstanding history of cough, sputum production, or shortness of breath as usual symptoms. Therefore, the first step is to determine whether the symptoms differ or are consistent with the individual's usual symptoms. This involves asking additional screening questions to assess whether the symptoms are stable, increased, or have changed over time compared to the usual symptoms. Failure to correctly classify these symptoms during determination of eligibility is one of the reasons for higher rates of positive screens than expected for LCS programs.

Primary care providers often acknowledge needing more guidance in determining screening eligibility for LDCT screening. This guidance is usually requested from specialists who are more knowledgeable in LCS. As a result, several LDCT programs have centralized the screening eligibility assessment, shared decision making (SDM) visit, and counseling on tobacco cessation. Centralized LDCT screening programs are specialist driven, with recruitment, SDM, and tobacco cessation counseling (TCC) performed by dedicated LCS personnel only [16, 17]. These programs require a referral to the program and are often led by an advanced licensed nurse practitioner (LNP) or LCS coordinator. The coordinator is responsible for contacting individuals referred to the program to determine their eligibility for LDCT screening, and conduct the SDM discussion. The LNP or LCS coordinator is usually the first point of contact for individuals referred to the LCS program. The coordinator confirms the individual meets eligibility requirements based on screening criteria set by payers and the individual's risk for lung cancer. They are responsible for ensuring that screenees have an understanding of the potential benefits and harms of screening. Individuals referred by PCPs are only scheduled for a LDCT screening scan after speaking with the LNP or LCS coordinator. The coordinator can also consult with clinicians, e.g., pulmonologists, in the LCS program to help determine the appropriateness of individuals for LDCT screening. To ensure risk for lung cancer, the coordinator performs a smoking pack-year calculation elicited from information provided by the individual, and includes consideration of previous quit attempts, length of quit, and determination of variability in numbers of cigarettes smoked [16]. This estimate is based on self-report bias and requires some calculation by providers, which may be challenged as guidelines for USPSTF and the CMS are slightly different [18–21]. Several pack-years calculations have been proposed for use in clinical practice including the one by Modine et al. in which pack-years is calculated using the average number of packs of cigarettes smoked per day × (age at time of referral − age became regular daily smoker − successful quit years) [16]. Once an individual is determined to meet criteria for LCS, the SDM and TCC visit is performed and an LDCT screening scan is ordered. Proponents of centralized LCS programs usually argue that the advantages to this structure include improvement in the efficiency and quality of the shared decision-making visit, screening implementation based on national standards, and improved tracking and care coordination of any findings on the screening study.

Nonetheless, recommendations provided by PCPs are shown to have a significant influence on patient screening behaviors [22]. PCPs are both essential and central to most LCS programs. In contrast to centralized programs, decentralized LDCT screening programs depend on PCPs to recruit and ensure eligibility of individuals for screening and then perform the required SDM and counseling on tobacco cessation prior to screening [23, 24]. However, in a single clinical visit, PCPs often have many considerations including management of acute and chronic illnesses, and preventive health services other than LDCT screening which can create competing interests. Yarnell et al. in their study found that PCPs with a practice of 2500 patients would have to spend more than 7 h per day to implement all of the preventive services recommended by the USPSTF [25]. Decision support tools, which assist PCPs in efficiently and effectively determining an individual's smoking history, age, and other requirements for LCS are essential.

PCPs also acknowledge the usefulness of EHR-based tools in alerting them to LDCT screening eligible patients [26, 27]. Support tools leveraging the power of

EHRs are effective in facilitating screening of potentially eligible patients. As discussed later in this chapter, one of the main advantages of EHRs is the collection and storage of clinical data, such as patient age and smoking status, which can later be queried [28, 29]. As age and smoking status are major components in LDCT screening eligibility criteria, EHRs are primed to help facilitate screening of potentially eligible patients in a systematic, high throughput manner. Triplette and colleagues demonstrated this potential in a cross-sectional cohort study of the National Health and Nutritional Examination Survey from 2011 to 2016 that included 235 million subjects [26]. Using simplified criteria of age and smoking status as a "pre-screening tool," the authors were able to effectively discriminate individuals who would ultimately be eligible for LDCT screening with a sensitivity of 100% and specificity of 88%. Notably, this simplified criteria did not require an assessment of pack-years [26]. This study highlights the potential of EHRs to serve as a first-pass screen to assess eligibility for LDCT screening across a patient cohort.

EHRs can also have the built-in functionality or be customizable to allow for integration of clinical decision support tools to provide real-time input in the assessment and confirmation of LDCT screening eligibility. These tools can include "flagging" of potentially eligible patients to prime PCPs regarding discussion of LDCT screening eligibility, as well as workflow prompts that can help confirm eligibility, facilitate appropriate documentation, and issue screening referrals. Implementation of these strategies has been successful in improving lung cancer screening rates in community practices. For example, Atrium Health, a community-based healthcare system serving approximately 1.1 million primary care patients, customized their EHR to systematically capture an extended smoking history including number of pack-years and quit date [30]. They also incorporated a health maintenance alert in the charts of patients meeting age and smoking criteria for LDCT screening based on their inputted data. Following implementation of these changes, quarterly LDCT screening referrals increased by 500% [30]. Although these findings support the use of clinical decision support tools reflecting best practices, such tools may not be ubiquitous to all primary care settings. A survey of 1384 PCPs from January 2014 to October 2015 found that only 11.2% of respondents had electronic reminders that notify them when a patient was due for LDCT screening assessment despite the vast majority of these respondents indicating that they use some form of EHR in their clinical practice [14]. Addressing this lack of availability of EHR-based support tools could significantly improve implementation of LCS.

EHRs are valuable in developing a systematic approach to screening and confirming patient eligibility for LDCT screening. However, the success of EHR-based solutions is contingent on having high-quality, accurate data that can be easily sorted and processed. In the 2016 study by Modin et al., pack-year discrepancies were found to exist between the EHR and shared decision making (SDM) consultation [16]. The authors showed that algorithms used by the EHR are still prone to inaccuracies and may continue to miss opportunities to screen-eligible adults [16]. Clinical data such as smoking pack-year history and quit date may not be routinely documented, accurately recorded, or adequately captured in EHRs. Inaccuracies in documentation can lead to either failure to recognize individuals eligible for screening, and, or performance of screening outside of eligibility guidelines. In a study on the implementation of LDCT screening in the Veterans Health Administration at eight different sites, 39.3% of identified patients had incomplete information regarding smoking status or incorrectly calculated pack-year history, rendering 36,555 persons ineligible for assessment for LDCT screening [31]. Other studies have also reported on concerns regarding documentation inaccuracies, with one survey study mentioning that only 29% of respondents would rely on their EHR data for making clinical decisions [16, 32]. Some LDCT screening programs use EHRs that do not identify smoking status in pack-years; and will require programming of the EHR to ask those questions that identify individuals as eligible for LCS. CMS documentation requirements mandate that EHRs should include appropriate templates for assessment of pack-year history [10]. Interventions specifically targeting improving smoking history documentation have been noted to improve LCS referral rates [26].

Institution of a navigator—nurse, midlevel providers, patient navigators—into a decentralized LDCT screening program is another highly effective solution to improve the assessment and confirmation of LCS eligibility. Furthermore, it allows for clear delineation of responsibilities, thereby streamlining the screening and confirmation process and improving overall LDCT screening efficiency. Percac-Lima and colleagues performed a randomized clinical trial assessing the impact of layperson navigators on LDCT screening rates and outcomes [33]. Navigator activities included taking a detailed smoking history to help assess if patients who were initially screened as having a history of smoking met the pack-year and time frame requirements of screening criteria. Navigators also assisted in education efforts, arranging shared decision-making appointments, setting up reminders that help to overcome barriers to screening and follow-up, and in some programs, coordinating care associated with findings on the LCS study. Of the patients who received navigator assistance, 92% of eligible patients had a diagnostic or screening chest CT scan within the study period [33]. On intention to treat analysis, there was nearly a threefold higher proportion (23.5% vs. 8.6%) of lung cancer screening CT scans performed within the study period [33]. Other studies have similarly found that nurse-led consultations are effective at determining specifics of smoking use for confirmation of eligibility [16, 34]. These findings supporting the utility of navigators in improving identification and enrollment of eligible patients are in line with recommendations on implementing lung cancer screening programs as stated in a joint statement from the American Thoracic Society and American College of Chest Physicians [35].

Increased collaboration and guidance between PCPs and screening radiology facilities can also help to ensure appropriate LDCT screening and minimize harms from LCS. Radiology departments bring a lot of experience from having developed breast cancer screening programs which have many of the same elements and operational issues as LCS [36]. In screening facilities, computed tomography (CT) schedulers and technicians often speak with individuals to ensure appropriate referral for screening. Radiology technicians are also responsible for reviewing all screening referral orders to the screening facility to determine if the individual meets criteria for a LDCT scan by the time of appointment. Individuals referred for

LDCT who do not meet criteria can have the LDCT referral order canceled by the screening facility. Radiology practices can also help in identifying and confirming LDCT screening eligibility by helping to secure institutional support for creating EHR tools to identify high-risk individuals for potential screening enrollment and distributing tobacco use questionnaires in outpatient PCP clinics [24].

4.1.3 Suggested Areas of Research

Research is needed on how best to assist primary care with ensuring that individuals eligible for LDCT screening are appropriately being referred for screening. Determining eligibility is essential to the process of screening and will require more targeted education of PCPs. While there is no universally standardized approach to these physician education programs to date, several professional societies, such as the American College of Chest Physicians, have developed courses to try to address this important need. Alternative educational opportunities include formalized lectures and group-based interactive learning sessions [24]. In addition, more research is needed on the applicability and practicality of using risk prediction modeling in clinical practice. Current risk prediction models used to determine eligibility are not practical for use in a busy primary care setting. Limitations to using these models include: the need for more extensive medical record data, blood or biomarkers testing, and the limited use to only specific patient-populations. Research focusing on integration of risk prediction models into the EHR, or as an EHR-based tool to improve the assessment of screening eligibility while remaining practical for population-based screening is much needed.

4.2 Barriers to Implementing Lung Cancer Screening (LCS) in Clinical Practice

Primary care is paramount in the identification of individuals eligible for cancer screening, follow-up of screening results, and coordination of downstream testing and treatment [37]. However, cancer screening is only a small fraction of the general preventive health services provided in primary care. Implementation of a new screening program presents a challenge to any clinical practice [38]. More specifically, implementing lung cancer screening (LCS) in primary care, compared with other types of cancer screening and preventative health services, requires concerted effort, in part because of the busy nature of primary care, and the complexity of the process [34].

Literature assessing the readiness of primary care clinics to implement LCS programs, have found that only 10% of respondents had LCS available in their practice [13]. This study suggested that high levels of uncertainty about LDCT, including the need for guidance about implementation and concerns about how screening would be integrated into EHR creates challenges to LCS implementation [28]. Identifying and addressing these practical needs in primary care is an important step prior to beginning LCS implementation. Currently there is no existing readiness assessment tool designed for LCS programs. Allen et al. have proposed adapting existing readiness assessment tools in primary care for use in LCS programs. One such tool is the Diabetes Care Coordination Assessment which considers five domains: organizational capacity, care coordination, clinical management, quality improvement, and infrastructure in measuring primary care clinic readiness to coordinate care for adult patients with diabetes [39]. The Consolidated Framework for Implementation Research (CFIR), which is described later in this section, has also been used to assess readiness for implementation of LCS programs.

Expert groups offer general guidance on implementation of LCS. Increasingly available guidance describe eligible patients and the components necessary for a high-quality screening program. However, operationalizing such guidance in practice is challenging [35]. Research assessing the low uptake of LDCT screening in clinical practice has been limited and mainly focused on examining the perceptions and understandings of LCS intentions among patients and providers along with examinations of the association between uptake and patient's sociodemographic characteristics [13, 40, 41]. However, beyond these individual-level factors, implementation challenges likely also affect screening uptake [28]. Findings from a pilot cross-sectional survey study of providers, staff, and administrators in radiology and primary care at a single Veterans Affairs Medical Center suggest that health professionals working in radiology have higher levels of readiness for change than those in primary care for implementing LCS [37]. Instead of selection bias, the authors concluded that the results of their study were likely due to more organizational barriers perceived in primary care, than in radiology. In this section, we focus on barriers to implementing LCS in primary care organizations and define these barriers using the CFIR framework.

4.2.1 Discussing Barriers to Implementation of LCS in Primary Care

Barriers to implementation may arise at multiple levels of healthcare delivery: the patient level, the group level, the organizational level, or the market (policy) level [42]. Research looking at the barriers and facilitators to implementing evidence-based interventions into real-world settings and the influence on outcomes shows that many interventions found to be effective in research often fail to translate into meaningful patient care outcomes in real-world settings [43]. Estimates indicate that two-thirds of organizations' efforts to implement change fail [44]. There are a number of theories and models that are used to study the barriers to effective implementation of evidence-based interventions. A wide range of studies have used the Consolidated Framework for Implementation Research (CFIR) to study cancer screening interventions in community clinics, federally qualified health centers (FHQCs), and other healthcare settings [45–47].

The CFIR is meta-theoretical, and includes constructs from a synthesis of existing theories and models to enable the examination of factors that may be encountered during implementation of an intervention into practice [43]. It comprises five major domains—the intervention, the context "inner and outer settings," the individuals involved, and the process by which implementation is accomplished—that interact in ways to influence implementation effectiveness [43]. A number of studies have used the CFIR framework to study cancer screening, and Allen et al. were the first to use this framework to analyze LCS implementation at two federally qualified health centers (FQHCs) [28]. Using the CFIR framework, the authors were able to analyze factors associated with effective implementation of LDCT screening at one site and barriers to implementation at the second site. In this section, we will use the CFIR framework to identify and discuss the barriers to implementing LCS in any primary care setting.

4.2.2   Lung Cancer Screening Is Complex and Costly

Implementing LCS in primary care can be challenging if the intervention (i.e., LDCT screening) is perceived as a poor fit. LCS is often viewed as a highly complex, multi-faceted, intervention that is difficult to implement and adapt to primary care settings. According to the CFIR framework, it is important to first consider how an intervention will be perceived and adapted to the setting in which it is being implemented prior to the implementation process [43]. Individuals involved in the planning process of implementing LCS are primarily responsible for demonstrating and communicating the advantages and importance of LCS screening to both staff and leadership. The return on investment should be clearly articulated to staff and leadership from the beginning of the process. Failure to demonstrate importance and adaptability of the intervention (LCS) in meeting the needs of primary care can result in ambiguity, low buy-in and ultimately incomplete implementation [28].

In 2017, the American Cancer Society conducted a 2-year pilot study at two federally qualified health centers (FQHCs). Each site partnered with a local American College of Radiology (ACR) accredited screening facility to implement LCS and referral programs at the sites [28]. One site was successful in creating and implementing the program while the other struggled to overcome significant implementation barriers. Of the many challenges faced by each site, one of the primary challenges was the complexity of actually performing LCS. An example of this is primary care settings that lack access to an electronic health record (EHR) system or do not have the ability to customize existing EHR systems for LCS. At these sites LCS is often performed manually. Without an EHR system, patient screening, request and tracking of screening referrals are done manually. This is a time-intensive approach to LCS that involves numerous steps, actions and hand-offs from several persons including the patient; and unintentionally builds more complexity into the referral process [28]. Errors can occur at any of these handoffs causing the process to fail and the intervention to be unsuccessful. Fail safe mechanisms are often designed and incorporated to ensure LCS occurs, and follow-up is scheduled in a timely manner. However, incorporation of these mechanisms usually requires the hiring of several new staff members—referral coordinator, a nurse, or medical assistant—which can increase the cost associated with performing LCS manually.

Most primary care settings however, utilize EHR systems to identify, screen, and refer eligible individuals for LCS. EHR systems however, can unintentionally build more complexity into the LCS and referral process, making LCS screening more difficult to implement. As discussed in the last section, eligibility for LCS is based on age, and smoking history. Eligible persons must have smoked for at least 30 pack-years, and former smokers must have quit less than 15 years before screening. However, the EHR has limitations in identifying all those who are eligible for LDCT screening [48, 49]. Although the smoking status—current, former, or never—is generally indicated in the EHR, details that are required to calculate pack-years are frequently absent [50]. Determining screening eligibility among former smokers is particularly challenging because of the frequent omission of quit dates. One study reported a 96.2% discordance between patient report and the EHR record of smoking history; and the underreporting of smoking history such that 54% of patients would have been erroneously deemed eligible if using EHR alone [16]. Inaccurate and insufficient EHR data hinders population-wide identification of eligible individuals, limiting the usefulness of clinical reminder systems and the ability to accurately determine the fraction of eligible patients screened or need to be screened in a community [2]. Such hindrance increases both the complexity and cost of implementing LCS in primary care. Additional resources, both financial and resource investments are required to ensure that individuals identified by an EHR system as eligible for LCS actually qualify for screening and more individuals who qualify for screening are not being missed.

Decentralized and hybrid programs often provide support in the form of EHR-based tools to perform LDCT screening, and radiology-generated recommendations for management of screen-detected abnormalities [24]. Decentralized programs, as described in the last section, are primary care-driven and depend on PCPs to identify eligible patients and then perform the required shared decision making (SDM) and tobacco cessation counseling (TCC) prior to screening [23]. Hybrid programs in contrast contain elements of both centralized programs (specialist-driven) and decentralized programs. An example of an EHR-driven BPA in LCS, is one that triggers on potentially eligible patients for screening during the primary care appointment, prompting the provider to perform an assessment, an action, an order, or all three themselves. Alternatively, the provider can choose to close the BPA without action [51]. If an EHR-driven BPA is not adaptable or customizable to the normal office workflow—e.g., changing the reminder to trigger during the assessment by a nurse—it is likely to be perceived as a poor fit in LCS implementation [43]. EHR-driven BPAs, as in the example above, can disrupt central workflow and processes by introducing several additional intervention steps in the LDCT screening process. This disruption can be burdensome, particularly to PCPs who screen for numerous conditions within time constrained visits.

The cost of implementing LDCT screening in primary care is not small. Mejia and colleagues in their survey of key informants reference lack of resources for LDCT screening as the most common barrier to implementing screening [52]. When considering cost, the cost of an intervention includes the financial and resource investments required to implement and sustain an intervention [28]. Since the advent of the US Preventive Services Task Force (USPSTF) certification and Centers for Medicare and Medicaid Services (CMS) approval, third party payment in the USA has become more common than offering LDCT screening services on a cash basis [4, 53–55]. Precertification may or may not be necessary depending on the payer [56]. However, many LCS programs will find that these direct reimbursement sources do not cover the entire cost of a LCS program [56]. In states with Medicaid expansion that reimburse LDCT screening, Medicaid and some private insurers will not reimburse follow-up tests done within certain months of the initial screening, despite ACR guidelines recommending follow-up after certain Lung-RADS findings [5]. Therefore to address these reimbursement errors, staff resources are allocated to engaging with insurance and reimbursement experts. Primary care considering implementing LCS programs in areas without Medicaid expansion, do not face reimbursement challenges; instead, such programs face the challenge of needing to identify funds up front to pay for screening and follow-up tests, once the program is implemented [28]. PCPs are required to have upfront knowledge of state reimbursement policies for LCS prior to the implementation process. Lack of knowledge of the differences in coverage policies can increase the burden and cost to primary care in implementing LCS.

The highest cost to primary care in implementing LCS is the resource investment. Resources have to be allocated to personnel—hospital administration, business management, marketing, clinical staff (nurse navigator, providers)—that oversee LCS; and to service coverage—medications for tobacco cessation, staff training, radiology and referral services, or access to LDCT—for LCS. Primary care settings without the staff and time to allocate to the LCS process will have challenges in implementing and sustaining LCS. Downstream investigations are often performed to follow up on LDCT scan findings before the next screening LDCT [57]. This is a high cost service coverage that can create challenges to implementing LCS in primary care and is discussed in more detail in Chap. 5.

4.2.3 External Influences Is a Barrier to Lung Cancer Screening Implementation

Implementation outcomes are impacted by: the networks and communication within the organization, the implementation climate, and the readiness of the organization to implement an LDCT program [28]. Networks and communication differ considerably within organizations. Regardless of the structure of an organization, the importance of communication across an organization is clear [43]. Direct and open communication for example, between a referring provider (PCP) and the screening facility or between leadership and clinical staff, is necessary throughout the LCS implementation process. Failure to engage in regular and open communication throughout the implementation process can lead to misunderstandings about the process, and lack of clarity about the goals and division of responsibilities within the program.

Individuals belonging to organizations with higher readiness of change are more likely to initiate change, and exert a greater effort to implement new evidence-based practices [58]. In contrast, primary care organizations that are facing competing priorities at the time of LCS implementation may struggle with leadership engagement. Implementation of a highly complex program such as LCS can be viewed as a low priority by organizations facing many competing priorities and with limitations on resources. Prioritization issues at the leadership level can also trickle down to the individual level [28]. Within an organization, individual roles are an important influencer on the success of implementing LCS. Roles and expectations for all staff involved in implementing LCS should be clearly delineated. Two key roles are "implementation leaders" and "champions" who serve as a bridge for communication and coordination between referring sites (PCP offices) and the screening facility or between leadership and staff [43]. Individuals are often nominated or appointed to these roles, with the expectation that implementing LCS is their sole top priority. However, an individual in this role, and facing competing priorities, for example, a referral coordinator serving multiple roles within a primary care clinic, is less likely to give the time and attention needed to implementing a LCS program. Engaging individuals tasked with implementing an intervention is often an overlooked part of implementation [59]. Individual-level barriers to implementing LCS are discussed in more detail in the sections on Shared Decision Making and Health Disparities in LCS.

4.2.4 Future Direction

More research is needed in readiness assessment tools specifically designed for implementing LCS in primary care. This assessment tool should include: identifying competing priorities, concurrent activities, ongoing or upcoming system challenges, and system readiness prior to the full implementation of the LCS program [28]. The higher levels of readiness for change found among radiology health professionals and self-identified leaders can be leveraged to develop strategies to engage PCPs with lower levels of readiness and lower value of change [37]. Future studies should focus on designing robust implementation strategies specifically for primary care. The findings from these studies should directly inform strategies on identifying eligible patients for LCS, conducting shared decision-making visits, resource allocation to managing abnormal screening results; and other challenges specific to primary care [31, 37, 39]. However, with thoughtful planning, open communication, and motivated individuals, [28] primary care can ultimately build a path to LCS and reducing LCS deaths.

4.3 Integration of Lung Cancer Screening into the Electronic Health Record

As lung cancer screening (LCS) programs proliferate in the decade since the publication of the National Lung Screening Trial, electronic health record (EHR) systems provide unique opportunities for improving efficiency and increasing scale [60]. The EHR, with its capacity for large-volume data capture and storage, can be used to improve multiple facets of the LCS process [61]. However, many health systems have been unable to optimize the strengths of the EHR, and in some cases the EHR can even hinder LCS. Limitations of the EHR can include inaccurate documentation of smoking history, non-standardized templates or procedure codes, non-discrete data entry which prevents data extraction, and exclusion of individuals—particularly vulnerable patients—who have not previously entered a health system or hospital for medical care. Despite these complexities at the health system or institutional level, for primary care providers (PCPs) the EHR is a valuable resource for identifying LCS-eligible individuals, documenting shared decision-making visits, tracking screen-detected lung nodules, and facilitating multidisciplinary evaluation for positive scans. Identification of strategies to leverage the EHR's strengths has significant potential to reduce barriers and improve LCS, as well as other population-based health interventions.

4.3.1 Areas of Focus for Leveraging the EHR

4.3.1.1 Documentation of Lung Cancer Risk Factors

As previously stated, inaccuracies in cigarette smoking history documentation are a well-known challenge in leveraging the EHR to determine LCS eligibility. Specific issues with smoking history documentation can include incomplete or inaccurate data entry by healthcare providers or ancillary staff. Additionally, software that updates smoking intensity by overwriting previous records presents a significant limitation. Data fields for comprehensive smoking history documentation are often suboptimal, including only years of smoking and packs per day, rather than also including start dates and cessation dates in an iterative fashion. Finally, LCS eligibility assessments based on smoking history must remain accurate even as eligibility guidelines undergo revision [15].

In one study, 96.2% of individuals referred to a centralized LCS program in Seattle had inaccurate pack-year history recorded in the EHR when compared with the smoking history elicited during shared decision making for LCS [16]. Of these, 85.2% of cases underreported smoking intensity, and the mean discordance was greater than 29 pack-years. Similarly, another group found that documentation of smoking years and intensity was missing or inaccurate in the EHR for more than half of individuals who participated in a pragmatic trial testing an LCS decision aid, with accurate pack-years documented for only 20% of participants [62]. These and other studies have demonstrated that based on EHR-available smoking history, only between 25% and 45% of individuals eligible for LCS would be correctly identified using EHR-derived cigarette smoking data [16, 62, 63]. Moreover, individuals with an erroneous EHR-recorded smoking history (despite clear previous documentation of LCS eligibility of 30 pack-years) were 33% less likely to have an LDCT ordered [64]. These studies demonstrate that reliance on EHR-derived smoking data may contribute to underscreening of individuals at high risk for lung cancer.

PCPs play a critical role in improving accuracy of recorded smoking history. One case study demonstrated that interventions such as training, process improvement, data management, and performance feedback were effective in improving smoking history documentation for lung cancer risk assessment in the EHR [65]. Process improvements included implementation of a population health dashboard for risk factor documentation and LCS rates across eight primary care clinics, and the sharing of best practices among participating sites. This quality improvement initiative demonstrates that primary care can drive foundational success for clinical components critical to LCS.

The extensive data storage capabilities of the EHR also provide an opportunity for capturing additional lung cancer risk factors such as the presence of COPD, family history of lung cancer, and occupational exposures, among others. Several lung cancer risk models in common use incorporate these factors [66, 67]. Wilshire and colleagues found that among individuals referred to an LCS program for screening with a COPD diagnostic term in their EHR record, 68% of these were actually an unsubstantiated diagnosis [68]. Although the National Comprehensive Cancer Network's Group II eligibility criteria for LCS (which included a clinical risk factor increasing lung cancer risk) are no longer in use, this provides another example of EHR inaccuracies which may have significant clinical impact on LCS utilization.

If these challenges can be overcome, a highly accurate EHR has the potential to advance LCS through a myriad of process improvements. At the health system level, patients eligible for LCS could be easily identified, thus facilitating patient conversations by primary care providers and more accurate referrals for screening.

Additionally, screen-eligible individuals who have current smoking status could be identified for more targeted tobacco treatment counseling efforts. Finally, more accurate EHR data would spur greater research efforts at the population level.

4.3.2 EHR Support for Identifying LCS-Eligible Individuals

Once the EHR contains accurate and complete patient-level data that can be used to determine LCS eligibility, software systems can be harnessed to develop strategies for promoting screening and optimizing workflows. This includes clinical decision support and nudges, and electronic referrals for screening, scheduling of shared decision-making appointments, and LDCT scans. For PCPs in particular, electronic nudges linked directly to a screening referral or order can provide critical time-saving support. In an ideal system, the EHR would provide an integrated workflow for identifying eligible patients and facilitating referrals and scheduling for centralized, decentralized, and hybrid programs. While anecdotal use of EHR tools such as Best Practice Advisories to notify clinicians of potential eligibility for LCS is common, to our knowledge there is no data measuring the impact of these interventions in LCS [60, 69]. Additionally, there is inconsistent use of the EHR for screening referrals and standardized templates or procedure codes, even among institutions within a single health system [70].

Although electronic tools for patient communication using the EHR can improve screening rates and patient decision support in other cancers, this is yet to be established for LCS [69, 71]. O'Brien and colleagues carried out a mixed methods comparative study of electronic or paper-based forms to identify LCS-eligible patients in primary care practices and found that uptake overall was low, underscoring the multiple patient- and provider-related barriers to screening [72]. Additionally, the authors noted that EHR software needs to link eligibility criteria to appointment information in order to be considered feasible. In a separate study, Begnaud and colleagues tested electronic LCS promotion among individuals who were identified to have previously smoked through the EHR. Of 99 individuals who received the electronic message offering screening, fewer than 20% of individuals read the message and responded with a complete smoking history [55]. Only half of these patients were eligible for LCS. These studies demonstrate that EHR-based workflows to identify eligible patients remain hampered by low uptake, inaccurate EHR data, and lack of integrated software systems.

4.3.3 Tracking LDCT Findings for Follow-Up

Once an LCS-eligible individual completes the shared decision-making visit and LDCT scan, tracking of screen-detected nodules to ensure appropriate adherence continues to be a challenge for many LCS programs. LDCT results in the form of

Lung-RADS categories can be entered as discrete data, allowing for systematic alerts for nodules that require surveillance. Optimally, these systems would also facilitate communication between patients and providers, and additionally provide clinical decision support for guideline-concordant lung nodule management. Nodule tracking software systems that are currently available are limited by labor-intensive manual data entry and lack of seamless integration with large EHR systems. In current practice, these obstacles may outweigh the potential benefits of automated nodule tracking. Several studies have demonstrated successful strategies for process improvements in tracking incidental lung nodules [73–78]. It remains to be seen whether these methods can be applied to the LCS arena and scaled up for use at the health system level.

Additional measurement of screening outcomes is complicated by unstructured and incomplete information stored in the EHR [79]. For example, incidental findings such as coronary artery calcifications, thyroid nodules, and hepatic and renal cysts are common on LDCT scans performed for LCS [80]. Although some of these findings may require further evaluation, they are inconsistently described and rarely recorded as discrete data [81]. Comprehensive EHR software should allow for accurate measurement of clinical metrics integral to providing high-quality LCS [82].

PCPs can individually implement nodule tracking through existing EHR systems by setting interval reminders and messages for follow-up scans. Additional strategies proposed in a mixed methods study of PCPs include automation of orders for follow-up tests, longitudinal tracking tools for interval imaging, and decision guides or even virtual consultations embedded in the EHR [83]. In this study, PCPs also described time constraints as the greatest barrier to lung nodule management. Additionally, overreliance on the EHR can lead to electronic alert fatigue, which may inadvertently exacerbate the burden on primary care. In healthcare systems with a centralized LCS program, the EHR can be utilized for efficient results communication with PCPs. The burden of nodule tracking can be removed from primary care by dedicated screening navigators who can provide tracking and management services. These approaches require clear communication strategies and established workflows between LCS programs and primary care to ensure that patients are neither lost to follow-up nor receive redundant care.

4.3.4 Research Gaps

A myriad of research gaps remain in defining the optimal use of the EHR for lung cancer screening. It is critical for clinicians, data scientists and bioinformaticians, and information technology specialists to collaborate as the field moves forward with more sophisticated electronic capabilities. Analogous to the process of evaluating the evidence for molecular biomarker use in lung cancer, EHR process improvements should be rigorously defined and then tested prospectively in iterative fashion across multiple programs and health systems [84]. Other novel strategies—for example integrating quantitative imaging features, clinical parameters, and genomic analyses through convolutional neural networks and other machine learning methods—may allow for discrimination of benign versus neoplastic nodules [85–87]. Finally, prioritization of research among vulnerable populations will be critical to leveraging the EHR for the ultimate goal of broadening LCS uptake and improving health equity. For instance, it is unclear how to identify individuals—often from underserved populations—who are not connected to a health system. These and other initiatives will require a collaborative approach with public health scientists and experts in community outreach.

On a larger scale, the EHR can be used to carry out population-level studies across multiple health systems. For example, Ritzwoller and colleagues estimated the impact of the USPSTF expanded eligibility criteria on 5 community-based healthcare settings using EHR-derived data from 34,528 individuals [88]. These and other studies demonstrate the potential of using large EHR-based datasets—which contain reliable, longitudinal, real-world populations—as a powerful platform to more accurately define clinical outcomes in lung cancer [89–91].

4.3.5 Future Directions

PCPs can leverage the EHR to facilitate LCS in decentralized programs while also providing critical support to centralized LCS programs through improvement of EHR documentation. On a larger scale, the EHR can be leveraged across the continuum of care in LCS to improve uptake, facilitate screening completion, and track adherence. EHR-derived data can also be utilized for population-level research on lung cancer outcomes. Therefore, defining and testing EHR-based strategies for LCS management will be a critical advance for the field. Moreover, collaboration between clinicians and bioinformaticians will be essential to develop seamless integration of LCS-specific software with existing EHRs. PCPs play an essential role in advocating for systems-level approaches to facilitating LCS, and input from primary care is critical to ensuring successful implementation of the LCS process. Only when these EHR-based workflows and analytical tools have been optimized can the field realize the promise of reducing mortality for all individuals at risk for lung cancer.

4.4 Insurance Coverage and Prior Authorization of Lung Cancer Screening

In 2022, most high-risk individuals with private or public health insurance will have coverage for low-dose CT (LDCT) scans for lung cancer screening (LCS) without cost-sharing. Notable exceptions are individuals with Medicaid residing in states that have opted against Medicaid expansion under the affordable care act (ACA) and have opted not to cover LCS, individuals with a small handful of private insurance plans which were in place prior to the passing of the ACA in 2010, and most individuals with short-term insurance plans. Prior authorization requirements and accepted International Classification of Diseases, Tenth Revision, Clinical Modification (ICD-10-CM) diagnosis codes may vary by plan. In addition, most plans are not required to cover services provided by out of network providers. It is important to note that coverage without cost-sharing generally applies only to yearly LDCT scans (and shared decision-making visits for patients with Medicare). Many patients will experience co-pays and cost-sharing for diagnostic CT scans and other tests ordered to evaluate abnormal findings identified through screening.

4.4.1 Private Insurance Coverage

In 2013, the United States Preventive Services Task Force (USPSTF) provided LCS with LDCT a grade B recommendation for adults ages 55–80 with at least a 30 pack-year smoking history who currently smoke or have quit within the past 15 years [4]. In March 2021, this recommendation was updated to include individuals ages 50–80 with at least a 20 pack-year smoking history who currently smoke and who have quit within the past 15 years [5]. It is recommended to stop screening if an individual develops a health condition that limits life expectancy or is unwilling to undergo curative treatment for lung cancer. Under the ACA, private insurance plans generally are required to provide coverage for all grade A and B rated preventative services without cost-sharing with a few notable exceptions [92]. A small number of private insurance plans which existed prior to the enactment of the ACA in 2010 are considered to have "grandfathered status" and are not subject to the ACA's requirements to cover preventive services [93]. Similarly, patients with "short-term" health plans generally do not have coverage for preventive care. For patients with these health plans, individual plan documents will need to be consulted to determine coverage and cost-sharing. For most patients with private group or individual health insurance, screening will be covered without cost-sharing. Prior authorization requirements and accepted ICD-10-CM diagnosis codes may vary by plan.

4.4.2 Medicare Coverage

In 2015, Centers for Medicare and Medicaid Services (CMS) issued a decision memo determining that there was sufficient evidence to justify coverage of LDCT scans for LCS for eligible beneficiaries [94]. LCS is now covered by Medicare Part B as well as by Medicare Advantage plans, which are plans offered by private insurance companies who contract with the federal government. CMS defined eligible beneficiaries as follows:

- Age 55–77 years
- Asymptomatic (no signs or symptoms of lung cancer)
- At least 30 pack-year smoking history
- Current smoker or one who has quit smoking within the last 15 years

In addition to the above criteria, the CMS decision included an unprecedented requirement that beneficiaries first undergo a lung cancer screening counseling and shared decision-making visit with a physician or qualified non-physician practitioner prior to the screening test being ordered. The shared decision-making visit is a face-to-face encounter required prior to the initial screen only and can be performed in person or via telehealth. Subsequent LCS studies do not require a shared decision-making visit, however, one may be conducted and billed for. Shared decision-making visits are billed for using the Current Procedural Terminology (CPT) code G0296 which must be linked to an appropriate ICD-10-CM diagnosis code for former (Z87.891) or current (F17.21*) nicotine dependence (see Table 4.2). The shared decision-making visit can be performed as part of an Evaluation and Management visit and billed using the 25 modifier. In order to qualify for coverage, the provider performing the shared decision-making visit must document the following elements in the patient's medical record:

Table 4.2 Common billing codes associated with lung cancer screening

	CPT Code	
Lung cancer screening CT scan	71271	Computed tomography, thorax, low dose for lung cancer screening without contrast material(s)
Shared decision-making visit	G0296	Counseling visit to discuss need for lung cancer screening using low-dose CT scan (LDCT)
Tobacco cessation counseling	99406	Smoking and tobacco use cessation counseling visit; intermediate, 3–10 min
	99407	Smoking and tobacco use cessation counseling visit; >10 min
	ICD-10-CM Code	
Former smokers	Z87.891	Personal history of tobacco use/personal history of nicotine dependence
Current smokers	F17.210	Nicotine dependence, cigarettes, uncomplicated
	F17.211	Nicotine dependence, cigarettes, in remission
	F17.213	Nicotine dependence, cigarettes, with withdrawal
	F17.218	Nicotine dependence, cigarettes, with other nicotine-induced disorders
	F17.219	Nicotine dependence, cigarettes, with unspecified nicotine-induced disorders

- Determination of beneficiary eligibility including age, absence of signs or symptoms of lung cancer, a specific calculation of cigarette smoking pack-years; and if a former smoker, the number of years since quitting.
- Shared decision making, including the use of one or more decision aids, to include benefits and harms of screening, follow-up diagnostic testing, over-diagnosis, false positive rate, and total radiation exposure.
- Counseling on the importance of adherence to annual lung cancer LDCT screening, impact of comorbidities and ability or willingness to undergo diagnosis and treatment.
- Counseling on the importance of maintaining cigarette smoking abstinence if former smoker; or the importance of smoking cessation if current smoker and, if appropriate, furnishing of information about tobacco cessation interventions.
- If appropriate, the furnishing of a written order for lung cancer screening with LDCT.

The order for both the initial and subsequent LCS LDCT scans must include the following information: the beneficiary date of birth, actual pack-year smoking history (number), current smoking status and for former smoker the number of years since quitting smoking, a statement that the beneficiary is asymptomatic and National Provider Identifier (NPI) of the ordering practitioner.

The appropriate CPT code for LDCT scans for LCS is 71271 "Computed tomography, thorax, low dose for lung cancer screening, without contrast material(s)." Unlike patients with commercial insurance, LDCT scans for LCS are not currently covered for patients with Medicare if they are performed in an Independent Diagnostic Testing Facility (IDTF).

4.4.3 Medicaid Coverage

Unlike Medicare, which is operated by the federal government, states operate their own Medicaid programs under broad federal guidelines. While federal law requires certain mandatory benefits to be covered, states have broad leeway to determine the scope of optional benefits provided. Under the ACA, states are given the option to expand Medicaid coverage to individuals who fall within 138% of the federal poverty level. States which elect to expand Medicaid must provide coverage without cost-sharing for all preventative services given a grade A or B rating from the USPSTF. This includes coverage for LCS for those who meet USPSTF eligibility criteria. In states that have not opted to expand Medicaid, states have the option to cover LCS but it is not required. As of January 2022, 39 states (including Washington DC) have opted to expand Medicaid [95]. For patients who reside in states without Medicaid expansion, coverage and eligibility may vary and will need to be researched prior to ordering a LCDT for LCS.

4.4.4 Prior Authorization

For patients with traditional Medicare (i.e., Medicare Part B), prior authorization is not required for coverage as long as the appropriate information is provided in the LCS LDCT order, and the order is associated with an accepted ICD-10-CM code. Patients with Medicare Advantage plans may require prior authorization. Similarly, prior authorization is commonly required for coverage through private insurance programs and Medicaid. As prior authorization requirements vary by plan, the individual plan materials must be consulted to determine the required documentation as well as the accepted ICD-10-CM diagnosis codes.

References

1. National Lung Screening Trial Research Team, Aberle DR, Berg CD, Black WC, Church TR, Fagerstrom RM, Galen B, Gareen IF, Gatsonis C, Goldin J, Gohagan JK, Hillman B, Jaffe C, Kramer BS, Lynch D, Marcus PM, Schnall M, Sullivan DC, Sullivan D, Zylak CJ. The National Lung Screening Trial: overview and study design. Radiology. 2011;258(1):243–53. https://doi.org/10.1148/radiol.10091808. Epub 2010 Nov 2. PMID: 21045183; PMCID: PMC3009383.
2. Armstrong K, Kim JJ, Halm EA, Ballard RM, Schnall MD. Using lessons from breast, cervical, and colorectal cancer screening to inform the development of lung cancer screening programs. Cancer. 2016;122(9):1338–42. https://doi.org/10.1002/cncr.29937. Epub 2016 Feb 29. PMID: 26929386; PMCID: PMC4840047.
3. Wood DE, Eapen GA, Ettinger DS, et al. NCCN clinical practice guidelines in oncology: lung cancer screening. Version 1, 2012. http://www.nccn.org/professionals/physician_gls/pdf/lung_screening.pdf. Accessed 9 Jan 2012.
4. Moyer VA, U.S. Preventive Services Task Force. Screening for lung cancer: U.S. Preventive Services Task Force recommendation statement. Ann Intern Med. 2014;160(5):330–8. https://doi.org/10.7326/M13-2771. PMID: 24378917.
5. US Preventive Services Task Force, Krist AH, Davidson KW, Mangione CM, Barry MJ, Cabana M, Caughey AB, Davis EM, Donahue KE, Doubeni CA, Kubik M, Landefeld CS, Li L, Ogedegbe G, Owens DK, Pbert L, Silverstein M, Stevermer J, Tseng CW, Wong JB. Screening for lung cancer: US Preventive Services Task Force Recommendation Statement. JAMA. 2021;325(10):962–70. https://doi.org/10.1001/jama.2021.1117. PMID: 33687470.
6. Harris RP, Sheridan SL, Lewis CL, Barclay C, Vu MB, Kistler CE, Golin CE, DeFrank JT, Brewer NT. The harms of screening: a proposed taxonomy and application to lung cancer screening. JAMA Intern Med. 2014;174(2):281–5. https://doi.org/10.1001/jamainternmed.2013.12745. Erratum in: JAMA Intern Med. 2014 Mar;174(3):484. PMID: 24322781.
7. USPSTF (U.S. Preventive Services Task Force). Modeling report: other supporting document for lung cancer: screening. 2013. https://www.uspreventiveservicestaskforce.org/Page/Document/modeling-report/lung-cancer-screening. Accessed 15 Jan 2022.
8. Brenner DR, Boffetta P, Duell EJ, Bickeböller H, Rosenberger A, McCormack V, Muscat JE, Yang P, Wichmann H-E, Brueske-Hohlfeld I, Schwartz AG, Cote ML, Tjønneland A, Friis S, Le Marchand L, Zhang Z-F, Morgenstern H, SzeszeniaDabrowska N, Lissowska J, Zaridze D, Rudnai P, Fabianova E, Foretova L, Janout V, Bencko V, Schejbalova M, Brennan P, Mates IN, Lazarus P, Field JK, Raji O, McLaughlin JR, Liu G, Wiencke J, Neri M, Ugolini D, Andrew AS, Lan Q, Hu W, Orlow I, Park BJ, Hung RJ. Previous lung diseases and lung cancer risk: a pooled analysis from the International Lung Cancer Consortium. Am J Epidemiol. 2012;176(7):573–85.

9. McKee BJ, Hashim JA, French RJ, McKee AB, Hesketh PJ, Lamb CR, Williamson C, Flacke S, Wald C. Experience with a CT screening program for individuals at high risk for developing lung cancer. J Am Coll Radiol. 2015;12(2):192–7. https://doi.org/10.1016/j.jacr.2014.08.002. Epub 2014 Aug 28. PMID: 25176498.

10. CMS (Centers for Medicare & Medicaid Services). Decision memo for screening for lung cancer with low dose computed tomography (LDCT) (cag-00439n). 2015. https://www.cms.gov/medicare-coverage-database/view/ncacal-decision-memo.aspx?proposed=N&NCAId=274. Accessed 12 Nov 2021.

11. Ersek JL, Eberth JM, McDonnell KK, Strayer SM, Sercy E, Cartmell KB, Friedman DB. Knowledge of, attitudes toward, and use of low-dose computed tomography for lung cancer screening among family physicians. Cancer. 2016;122(15):2324–31.

12. Lewis JA, Petty WJ, Tooze JA, Miller DP, Chiles C, Miller AA, Bellinger C, Weaver KE. Low-dose CT lung cancer screening practices and attitudes among primary care providers at an academic medical center. Cancer Epidemiol Biomark Prev. 2015;24(4):664–70.

13. Volk RJ, Foxhall LE. Readiness of primary care clinicians to implement lung cancer screening programs. Prev Med Rep. 2015;2:717–9.

14. Raz DJ, Wu GX, Consunji M, Nelson R, Sun C, Erhunmwunsee L, et al. Perceptions and utilization of lung cancer screening among primary care physicians. J Thorac Oncol. 2016;11(11):1856–62.

15. Force UPST. Screening for lung cancer: US Preventive Services Task Force Recommendation Statement. JAMA. 2021;325(10):962–70.

16. Modin HE, Fathi JT, Gilbert CR, Wilshire CL, Wilson AK, Aye RW, Farivar AS, Louie BE, Vallieres E, Gorden JA. Pack year cigarette smoking history for determination of lung cancer screening eligibility. Comparison of the electronic medical record versus a shared decision-making conversation. Ann Am Thorac Soc. 2017;14:1320–5.

17. Mazzone PJ, Tenenbaum A, Seeley M, Petersen H, Lyon C, Han X, Wang XF. Impact of a lung cancer screening counseling and shared decision-making visit. Chest. 2017;151(3):572–8. https://doi.org/10.1016/j.chest.2016.10.027. Epub 2016 Nov 1. PMID: 27815154.

18. Paige SR, Salloum RG, Carter-Harris L. Assessment of lung cancer screening eligibility on NCI-designated cancer center websites. J Cancer Educ. 2021. https://doi.org/10.1007/s13187-021-02051-w. Epub ahead of print. PMID: 34478042.

19. US Preventive Services Task Force. Final recommendation statement: lung cancer: screening. https://www.uspreventiveservicestaskforce.org/Page/Document/RecommendationStatementFinal/lung-cancer-screening. Accessed 28 Jan 2022.

20. Jensen TS, Chin J, Ashby L, Hermansen J, Hutter JD. Decision memo for screening for lung cancer with low dose computed tomography (LDCT). 2015. https://www.cms.gov/medicare-cover age-database/details/nca-decision-memo.aspx?NCAId=274. Accessed 28 Jan 2022.

21. Kanodra NM, Pope C, Halbert CH, Silvestri GA, Rice LJ, Tanner NT. Primary care provider and the patient perspectives on lung cancer screening: a qualitative study. Ann Am Thorac Soc. 2016;13:1977–82.

22. Zapka JG, Lemon SC. Interventions for patients, providers, and health care organizations. Cancer. 2004;101:1165–87.

23. Janssen K, Schertz K, Rubin N, Begnaud A. Incidental findings in a decentralized lung cancer screening program. Ann Am Thorac Soc. 2019;16(9):1198–201. https://doi.org/10.1513/AnnalsATS.201812-908RL. [PubMed: 31251089].

24. Hirsch EA, New ML, Brown SL, Barón AE, Sachs PB, Malkoski SP. Impact of a hybrid lung cancer screening model on patient outcomes and provider behavior. Clin Lung Cancer. 2020;21(6):e640–6. https://doi.org/10.1016/j.cllc.2020.05.018. Epub 2020 May 23. PMID: 32631782; PMCID: PMC7606309.

25. Yarnall KSH, Pollak KI, Østbye T, Krause KM, Michener JL. Primary care: is there enough time for prevention? Am J Public Health. 2003;93(4):635–41.

26. Triplette M, Kross EK, Mann BA, Elmore JG, Slatore CG, Shahrir S, Romine PE, Frederick PD, Crothers K. An assessment of primary care and pulmonary provider perspectives on

lung cancer screening. Ann Am Thorac Soc. 2018;15(1):69–75. https://doi.org/10.1513/AnnalsATS.201705-392OC. PMID: 28933940; PMCID: PMC5822418.

27. Gestalter YB, Koppelman E, Bolton R, Slatore CG, Yoon SH, Cain HC, Tanner NT, Au DH, Clark JA, Wiener RS. Evaluations of implementation at early-adopting lung cancer screening programs: lessons learned. Chest. 2017;152(1):70–80. https://doi.org/10.1016/j.chest.2017.02.012. Epub 2017 Feb 20. PMID: 28223153.

28. Allen CG, Cotter MM, Smith RA, Watson L. Successes and challenges of implementing a lung cancer screening program in federally qualified health centers: a qualitative analysis using the Consolidated Framework for Implementation Research. Transl Behav Med. 2020;11(5):1088–98.

29. Ortmeyer K, Ma GX, Kaiser LR, Erkmen C. Effective educational approaches to training physicians about lung cancer screening. J Cancer Educ. 2022;37(1):52–7.

30. Doty J, Lackey L, Ersek J, Howard D, Clary A. P3.11-05 use of electronic medical record (EMR)-embedded clinical decision support tools improves lung cancer screening rates. J Thorac Oncol. 2018;13(10):S960.

31. Kinsinger LS, Anderson C, Kim J, Larson M, Chan SH, King HA, et al. Implementation of lung cancer screening in the veterans health administration. JAMA Intern Med. 2017;177(3):399–406.

32. Zeliadt SB, Hoffman RM, Birkby G, Eberth JM, Brenner AT, Reuland DS, et al. Challenges implementing lung cancer screening in federally qualified health centers. Am J Prev Med. 2018;54(4):568–75.

33. Percac-Lima S, Ashburner JM, Rigotti NA, Park ER, Chang Y, Kuchukhidze S, et al. Patient navigation for lung cancer screening among current smokers in community health centers a randomized controlled trial. Cancer Med. 2018;7(3):894–902.

34. Brenner AT, Cubillos L, Birchard K, Doyle-Burr C, Eick J, Henderson L, et al. Improving the implementation of lung cancer screening guidelines at an academic primary care practice. J Healthc Qual. 2018;40(1):27–35.

35. Wiener RS, Gould MK, Arenberg DA, Au DH, Fennig K, Lamb CR, et al. An official American Thoracic Society/American College of Chest Physicians policy statement: implementation of low-dose computed tomography lung cancer screening programs in clinical practice. Am J Respir Crit Care Med. 2015;192(7):881–91.

36. National Academies of Sciences, Engineering, and Medicine. Implementation of lung cancer screening: proceedings of a workshop. Washington, DC: The National Academies Press; 2017. https://doi.org/10.17226/23680.

37. Spalluto LB, Lewis JA, Stolldorf D, Yeh VM, Callaway-Lane C, Wiener RS, Slatore CG, Yankelevitz DF, Henschke CI, Vogus TJ, Massion PP, Moghanaki D, Roumie CL. Organizational readiness for lung cancer screening: a cross-sectional evaluation at a Veterans Affairs Medical Center. J Am Coll Radiol. 2021;18(6):809–19. https://doi.org/10.1016/j.jacr.2020.12.010. Epub 2021 Jan 7. Erratum in: J Am Coll Radiol. 2021 Sep;18(9):1371. PMID: 33421372; PMCID: PMC8180484.

38. Erkmen CP, Moore RF, Belden C, DiSesa V, Kaiser LR, Ma GX, Paranjape A. Overcoming barriers to lung cancer screening by implementing a single-visit patient experience. Int J Cancer Oncol. 2017;4(2). https://doi.org/10.15436/2377-0902.17.1469. Epub 2017 May 17. PMID: 29399636; PMCID: PMC5796669.

39. McKee BJ, McKee AB, Flacke S, et al. Initial experience with a free, high-volume, low-dose CT lung cancer screening program. J Am Coll Radiol. 2013;10:586–92.

40. Carter-Harris L, Ceppa DP, Hanna N, Rawl SM. Lung cancer screening: what do long-term smokers know and believe? Health Expect. 2017;20(1):59–68. https://doi.org/10.1111/hex.12433. Epub 2015 Dec 23. PMID: 26701339; PMCID: PMC4919238.

41. Tanner NT, Egede LE, Shamblin C, Gebregziabher M, Silvestri GA. Attitudes and beliefs toward lung cancer screening among US Veterans. Chest. 2013;144(6):1783–7. https://doi.org/10.1378/chest.13-0056. PMID: 23764896; PMCID: PMC3848465.

42. Ferlie EB, Shortell SM. Improving the quality of health care in the United Kingdom and the United States: a framework for change. Milbank Q. 2001;79(2):281–315. https://doi.org/10.1111/1468-0009.00206. PMID: 11439467; PMCID: PMC2751188.

43. Damschroder LJ, Aron DC, Keith RE, Kirsh SR, Alexander JA, Lowery JC. Fostering implementation of health services research findings into practice: a consolidated framework for advancing implementation science. Implement Sci. 2009;4:50. https://doi.org/10.1186/1748-5908-4-50. PMID: 19664226; PMCID: PMC2736161.

44. Burnes B. Emergent change and planned change–competitors or allies?: The case of XYZ construction. Int J Oper Prod Manag. 2004;24(9):886–902. https://doi.org/10.1108/01443570410552108

45. Liang S, Kegler MC, Cotter M, Emily P, Beasley D, Hermstad A, Morton R, Martinez J, Riehman K. Integrating evidence-based practices for increasing cancer screenings in safety net health systems: a multiple case study using the Consolidated Framework for Implementation Research. Implement Sci. 2016;11:109. https://doi.org/10.1186/s13012-016-0477-4. Erratum in: Implement Sci. 2016;11(1):130. PMID: 27485452; PMCID: PMC4970264.

46. Walker TJ, Risendal B, Kegler MC, Friedman DB, Weiner BJ, Williams RS, Tu SP, Fernandez ME. Assessing levels and correlates of implementation of evidence-based approaches for colorectal cancer screening: a cross-sectional study with federally qualified health centers. Health Educ Behav. 2018;45(6):1008–15. https://doi.org/10.1177/1090198118778333. Epub 2018 Jul 10. PMID: 29991294; PMCID: PMC6226355.

47. Kegler MC, Liang S, Weiner BJ, Tu SP, Friedman DB, Glenn BA, Herrmann AK, Risendal B, Fernandez ME. Measuring constructs of the consolidated framework for implementation research in the context of increasing colorectal cancer screening in federally qualified health center. Health Serv Res. 2018;53(6):4178–203. https://doi.org/10.1111/1475-6773.13035. Epub 2018 Sep 10. PMID: 30260471; PMCID: PMC6232399.

48. Chen LH, Quinn V, Xu L, Gould MK, Jacobsen SJ, Koebnick C, Reynolds K, Hechter RC, Chao CR. The accuracy and trends of smoking history documentation in electronic medical records in a large managed care organization. Subst Use Misuse. 2013;48(9):731–42. https://doi.org/10.3109/10826084.2013.787095. Epub 2013 Apr 26. PMID: 23621678.

49. Wu YC, Perkovich MT, Woldemichael KM, et al. Electronic medical record smoking history does not accurately identify candidates for lung cancer screening—disproportionately affecting vulnerable and high-risk populations. Am J Respir Crit Care Med. 2016;193:A1092.

50. Begnaud AL, Joseph AM, Lindgren BR. Randomized electronic promotion of lung cancer screening: a pilot. JCO Clin Cancer Inform. 2017;1:1–6. https://doi.org/10.1200/CCI.17.00033. PMID: 30657381; PMCID: PMC6874003.

51. Kawamoto K, Houlihan CA, Balas EA, Lobach DF. Improving clinical practice using clinical decision support systems: a systematic review of trials to identify features critical to success. BMJ. 2005;330(7494):765. https://doi.org/10.1136/bmj.38398.500764.8F. Epub 2005 Mar 14. PMID: 15767266; PMCID: PMC555881.

52. Mejia MC, Zoorob R, Gonzalez S, Mosqueda M, Levine R. Key informants' perspectives on implementing a comprehensive lung cancer screening program in a safety net healthcare system: leadership, successes, and barriers. J Cancer Educ. 2021. https://doi.org/10.1007/s13187-020-01931-x. Epub ahead of print. PMID: 33417096.

53. Quaife SL, Marlow LAV, McEwen A, Janes SM, Wardle J. Attitudes towards lung cancer screening in socioeconomically deprived and heavy smoking communities: informing screening communication. Health Expect. 2017;20(4):563–73. https://doi.org/10.1111/hex.12481. Epub 2016 Jul 11. PMID: 27397651; PMCID: PMC5513004.

54. Rankin NM, McWilliams A, Marshall HM. Lung cancer screening implementation: complexities and priorities. Respirology. 2020;25(Suppl 2):5–23. https://doi.org/10.1111/resp.13963. PMID: 33200529.

55. http://www.cms.gov/medicare-coverage-database/details/nca-proposed-decision-memo.aspx?NCAId=274. Accessed 12 Nov 2021.

56. Optican RJ, Chiles C. Implementing lung cancer screening in the real world: opportunity, challenges and solutions. Transl Lung Cancer Res. 2015;4(4):353–64. https://doi.org/10.3978/j.issn.2218-6751.2015.07.14. PMID: 26380176; PMCID: PMC4549464.

57. Cressman S, Lam S, Tammemagi MC, Evans WK, Leighl NB, Regier DA, Bolbocean C, Shepherd FA, Tsao MS, Manos D, Liu G, Atkar-Khattra S, Cromwell I, Johnston MR, Mayo JR, McWilliams A, Couture C, English JC, Goffin J, Hwang DM, Puksa S, Roberts H, Tremblay A, MacEachern P, Burrowes P, Bhatia R, Finley RJ, Goss GD, Nicholas G, Seely JM, Sekhon HS, Yee J, Amjadi K, Cutz JC, Ionescu DN, Yasufuku K, Martel S, Soghrati K, Sin DD, Tan WC, Urbanski S, Xu Z, Peacock SJ; Pan-Canadian Early Detection of Lung Cancer Study Team. Resource utilization and costs during the initial years of lung cancer screening with computed tomography in Canada. J Thorac Oncol. 2014;9(10):1449–58. https://doi.org/10.1097/JTO.0000000000000283. PMID: 25105438; PMCID: PMC4165479.

58. Weiner BJ, Lewis MA, Linnan LA. Using organization theory to understand the determinants of effective implementation of worksite health promotion programs. Health Educ Res. 2009;24(2):292–305. https://doi.org/10.1093/her/cyn019. Epub 2008 May 9. PMID: 18469319.

59. Pronovost PJ, Berenholtz SM, Needham DM. Translating evidence into practice: a model for large scale knowledge translation. BMJ. 2008;337:a1714. https://doi.org/10.1136/bmj.a1714. PMID: 18838424.

60. Fathi JT, White CS, Greenberg GM, Mazzone PJ, Smith RA, Thomson CC. The integral role of the electronic health record and tracking software in the implementation of lung cancer screening; a call to action to developers: a white paper from the National Lung Cancer Roundtable. Chest. 2020;157(6):1674–9.

61. Hernandez-Boussard T, Blayney DW, Brooks JD. Leveraging digital data to inform and improve quality cancer care. Cancer Epidemiol Biomarkers Prev. 2020;29(4):816.

62. Patel N, Miller DP, Snavely AC, Bellinger C, Foley KL, Case D, et al. A comparison of smoking history in the electronic health record with self-report. Am J Prev Med. 2020;58(4):591–5.

63. Cole AM, Pflugeisen B, Schwartz MR, Miller SC. Cross sectional study to assess the accuracy of electronic health record data to identify patients in need of lung cancer screening. BMC Res Notes. 2018;11(1):14.

64. Tarabichi Y, Kats DJ, Kaelber DC, Thornton JD. The impact of fluctuations in pack-year smoking history in the electronic health record on lung cancer screening practices. Chest. 2018;153(2):575–8.

65. Peterson E, Harris K, Farjah F, Akinsoto N, Marcotte LM. Improving smoking history documentation in the electronic health record for lung cancer risk assessment and screening in primary care: a case study. Healthcare. 2021;9(4):100578.

66. Bach PB, Kattan MW, Thornquist MD, Kris MG, Tate RC, Barnett MJ, et al. Variations in lung cancer risk among smokers. J Natl Cancer Inst. 2003;95(6):470–8.

67. Tammemagi MC, Katki HA, Hocking WG, Church TR, Caporaso N, Kvale PA, et al. Selection criteria for lung-cancer screening. N Engl J Med. 2013;368(8):728–36.

68. Wilshire CL, Fuller CC, Gilbert CR, Handy JR, Costas KE, Louie BE, et al. Electronic medical record inaccuracies: multicenter analysis of challenges with modified lung cancer screening criteria. Can Respir J. 2020;2020:7142568.

69. Patel MS, Navathe AS, Liao JM. Using nudges to improve value by increasing imaging-based cancer screening. J Am Coll Radiol. 2020;17(1):38–41.

70. Gould MK, Sakoda LC, Ritzwoller DP, Simoff MJ, Neslund-Dudas CM, Kushi LH, et al. Monitoring lung cancer screening use and outcomes at four cancer research network sites. Ann Am Thorac Soc. 2017;14(12):1827–35.

71. Mougalian SS, Gross CP, Hall EK. Text messaging in oncology: a review of the landscape. JCO Clin Cancer Inform. 2018;2:1–9.

72. O'Brien MA, Sullivan F, Carson A, Siddiqui R, Syed S, Paszat L. Piloting electronic screening forms in primary care: findings from a mixed methods study to identify patients eligible for low dose CT lung cancer screening. BMC Fam Pract. 2017;18(1):95.

73. Weinstock TG, Tewari A, Patel H, Kelley K, Tananbaum R, Flores A, et al. No stone unturned: Nodule Net, an intervention to reduce loss to follow-up of lung nodules. Respir Med. 2019;157:49–51.
74. Lim PS, Schneider D, Sternlieb J, Taupin M, Sich N, Dian J, et al. Process improvement for follow-up radiology report recommendations of lung nodules. BMJ Open Qual. 2019;8(2):e000370.
75. Murphy DR, Thomas EJ, Meyer AND, Singh H. Development and validation of electronic health record–based triggers to detect delays in follow-up of abnormal lung imaging findings. Radiology. 2015;277(1):81–7.
76. Dyer DS, Zelarney PT, Carr LL, Kern EO. Improvement in follow-up imaging with a patient tracking system and computerized registry for lung nodule management. J Am Coll Radiol. 2021;18(7):937–46.
77. Aase A, Fabbrini AE, White KM, Averill S, Gravely A, Melzer AC. Implementation of a standardized template for reporting of incidental pulmonary nodules: feasibility, acceptability, and outcomes. J Am Coll Radiol. 2020;17(2):216–23.
78. Shelver J, Wendt CH, McClure M, Bell B, Fabbrini AE, Rector T, et al. Effect of an automated tracking registry on the rate of tracking failure in incidental pulmonary nodules. J Am Coll Radiol. 2017;14(6):773–7.
79. Rai A, Doria-Rose VP, Silvestri GA, Yabroff KR. Evaluating lung cancer screening uptake, outcomes, and costs in the united states: challenges with existing data and recommendations for improvement. J Natl Cancer Inst. 2019;111(4):342–9.
80. Morgan L, Choi H, Reid M, Khawaja A, Mazzone PJ. Frequency of incidental findings and subsequent evaluation in low-dose computed tomographic scans for lung cancer screening. Ann Am Thorac Soc. 2017;14(9):1450–6.
81. Mazzone PJ, Silvestri GA, Souter LH, Caverly TJ, Kanne JP, Katki HA, et al. Screening for lung cancer: CHEST guideline and expert panel report. Chest. 2021;160(5):e427–94.
82. Mazzone PJ, White CS, Kazerooni EA, Smith RA, Thomson CC. Proposed Quality Metrics for Lung Cancer Screening Programs: A National Lung Cancer Roundtable Project. Chest. 2021;160(1):368–78.
83. Talutis SD, Childs E, Goldman AL, Knapp PE, Gupta A, Ferrao C, et al. Strategies to optimize management of incidental radiographic findings in the primary care setting: a mixed methods study. Am J Surg. 2022;223(2):297–302.
84. Mazzone PJ, Sears CR, Arenberg DA, Gaga M, Gould MK, Massion PP, et al. Evaluating molecular biomarkers for the early detection of lung cancer: when is a biomarker ready for clinical use? An Official American Thoracic Society Policy Statement. Am J Respir Crit Care Med. 2017;196(7):e15–29.
85. Baldwin DR, Gustafson J, Pickup L, Arteta C, Novotny P, Declerck J, et al. External validation of a convolutional neural network artificial intelligence tool to predict malignancy in pulmonary nodules. Thorax. 2020;75(4):306.
86. Massion PP, Antic S, Ather S, Arteta C, Brabec J, Chen H, et al. Assessing the accuracy of a deep learning method to risk stratify indeterminate pulmonary nodules. Am J Respir Crit Care Med. 2020;202(2):241–9.
87. Wang J, Gao R, Huo Y, Bao S, Xiong Y, Antic SL, et al. Lung cancer detection using co-learning from chest CT images and clinical demographics. In: Proceedings of SPIE—the International Society for Optical Engineering; 2019 (0277-786X (Print)).
88. Ritzwoller DP, Meza R, Carroll NM, Blum-Barnett E, Burnett-Hartman AN, Greenlee RT, et al. Evaluation of population-level changes associated with the 2021 US Preventive Services Task Force lung cancer screening recommendations in community-based health care systems. JAMA Netw Open. 2021;4(10):e2128176-e.
89. Yuan Q, Cai T, Hong C, Du M, Johnson BE, Lanuti M, et al. Performance of a machine learning algorithm using electronic health record data to identify and estimate survival in a longitudinal cohort of patients with lung cancer. JAMA Netw Open. 2021;4(7):e2114723-e.

90. Carr LL, Zelarney P, Meadows S, Kern JA, Long MB, Kern E. Development of a cancer care summary through the electronic health record. J Oncol Pract. 2016;12(2):e231–e40.
91. Yeh MA-O, Wang YA-O, Yang HA-O, Bai KA-O, Wang HA-O, Li YA-O. Artificial intelligence-based prediction of lung cancer risk using nonimaging electronic medical records: deep learning approach. J Med Internet Res. 2021;23(8)(1438-8871 (Electronic)).
92. Seiler N, MalCarney M, et al. Coverage of clinical preventive services under the affordable care act: from law to access. Public Health Rep. 2014;129(6):526–32.
93. Internal Revenue Service, Department of the Treasury; Employee Benefits Security Administration, Department of Labor; Office of Consumer Information and Insurance Oversight, Department of Health and Human Services. Interim final rules for group health plans and health insurance coverage relating to status as a grandfathered health plan under the Patient Protection and Affordable Care Act. Interim final rules with request for comments. Fed Regist. 2010;75(116):34537–70.
94. Centers for Medicare & Medicaid Services. Decision memo for screening for lung cancer with low dose computed tomography (LDCT) (CAG-00439N). Published February 2015. https://www.cms.gov/medicare-coverage-database/view/ncacal-decision-memo.aspx?proposed=N&NCAId=274. Accessed 27 Jan 2022.
95. Kaiser Family Foundation. Status of state medicaid expansion decisions: interactive map. Updated January 18, 2022. https://www.kff.org/medicaid/issue-brief/status-of-state-medicaid-expansion-decisions-interactive-map/. Accessed 27 Jan 2022.

Chapter 5
Innovations in Integrating Smoking Cessation and the Shared Decision-Making Discussion into Lung Cancer Screening

Theresa Roelke, Richard M. Schwartzstein, Thomas Houston, and Douglas Holt

Lung cancer survival is expected to double by 2025 in part through increased low-dose computed tomography (LDCT) screening for early detection. The lung screening process begins with a shared decision-making (SDM) discussion between a clinician, who could be a primary care physician (PCP) or an individual with experience and expertise in lung cancer screening, and a patient to decide whether or not to pursue lung cancer screening. The consult is meant to address risks and benefits of cancer screening, false positive and false negative findings, smoking cessation and the uncertainty associated with discovery of pulmonary nodules, and address the impact of comorbidities such as emphysema and atherosclerosis on the thought process about screening.

This chapter discusses SDM within the context of LCS. Additionally, we look toward the future of LCS, which will incorporate innovative tools to engage patients visually while creating an experiential learning environment designed to reduce anxiety, through improved understanding of pulmonary nodules and the screening process, and to enhance support for smoking cessation.

T. Roelke (✉)
MaineHealth, Maine Medical Center, Maine Medical Center Research Institute, Maine Medical Partners, Scarborough, ME, USA
e-mail: Theresa.Roelke@MaineHealth.com

R. M. Schwartzstein
Division of Pulmonary, Critical Care and Sleep Medicine, Beth Israel Deaconess Medical Center, Harvard Medical School, Boston, MA, USA

T. Houston
Department of Family and Community Medicine, The Ohio State University College of Medicine, Columbus, OH, USA

D. Holt
Idaho Cancer Center, Radiation Oncology, Idaho Falls, ID, USA

© The Author(s), under exclusive license to Springer Nature Switzerland AG 2022
J. V. Baptiste et al. (eds.), *Lung Cancer Screening*,
https://doi.org/10.1007/978-3-031-10662-0_5

5.1   Components of a Shared Decision-Making Discussion

SDM occurs every day in business, education, and in healthcare where it is at the heart of quality, patient-centered care and a key component of every conversation conducted with patients and families about their own healthcare or the care of a loved one. SDM is a mindful process in which a healthcare provider, patient, and family discuss, collaborate on and determine an overall plan of care for maintaining good health and quality of life consistent with the patient's goals and values in light of their unique lifestyle and family setting.

During a SDM discussion for LCS, a clinician reviews clinical evidence with an eligible patient to ensure LCS aligns with the patient's personal values and preferences and, consequently, that the decision to screen is right for them.

Components of a LCS discussion include review of lung cancer screening criteria, a patient's risk of developing lung cancer, personal preferences, as well as the benefits or harms and comorbidities that may preclude additional diagnostics should a suspicious lesion be identified. A patient's functional status is reviewed as it relates to their willingness or ability to undergo treatment and/or curative surgery should they be diagnosed with lung cancer. Potential harms such as false negative results, false positive results and associated follow-up tests, incidental findings such as atherosclerosis and emphysema, and the potential for additional radiation exposure are also discussed. The risk of anxiety associated with inconclusive results is also considered as well as the burden of costs associated with additional testing not covered or fully reimbursed by insurance [1].

Benefits of LCS, including early detection, the reduction in lung cancer and all-cause mortality, and interventions for other findings on LDCT screening are important components of a SDM visit. Support for smoking cessation is offered through a variety of support systems including behavioral and pharmacotherapy, group programs, and tobacco helpline referrals are reviewed.

Decision Aids   Decision aids can be helpful tools to support the SDM discussion. Many decision aids or decision support tools have been developed to assist the provider. These paper-based, video, or web-based tools assist patients when evaluating their options. They may describe eligibility criteria, define key terms, show relevant anatomy, outline the timeline for CT scans, and delineate risks and benefits of the screening program. Trials of decision aids found patients become more engaged in the SDM process with the support of visual tools with a tendency to make mindful decisions [2]. Furthermore, they may assist clinicians who report they seldom offer the amount of information needed to allow patients to be fully engaged in shared decision-making for a lung nodule finding [3]. These tools may invite patients to become visually engaged in the discussion, which enhances their level of understanding, or they may lead to greater trust in the information shared by the provider.

In a 2020 study across 13 states, patients who met eligibility criteria for lung screening were selected through tobacco quitlines and randomized to the lung cancer screening video, "Is it right for me?" compared to standard of care. The study found that 67.4% who viewed the video were well-prepared to make a lung screening decision compared to 48.2% assigned to usual care. Fifty percent reported feeling informed about their decision with the assistance of the video compared with 28.3% in the standard of care cohort, and 68.0% felt confident and clear about their personal values as they related to risk and benefit of lung screening. Overall, participants exposed to the lung cancer screening shared decision-making video were more knowledgeable about lung screening than participants receiving usual care [4].

Decision aids can be cost effective during a SDM consultation. A randomized 2013 study of decision-making about medical treatment compared usual care to care with enhanced support, which included contact with trained health coaches via phone, mail, e-mail, and use of the internet. Patients who received enhanced support had 5.3% reduced medical costs than patients receiving usual care. The enhanced cohort had 12.5% fewer hospitalizations and 9.9 fewer preference-sensitive surgeries, many of which were cardiac surgeries. This type of remote or virtual models of support may be particularly effective for reaching rural communities, which comprise approximately 20% of the US population [5].

5.2 Challenges in Shared Decision-Making Decisions: Embracing Uncertainty

Since the report of the National Lung Cancer Screening Trial (NLST) [6], it has become clear that LDCT scan screening for lung cancer can save lives. Nonetheless, there are well-known downsides or risks to patients who participate in these programs including exposure to radiation, complications from procedures related to false positive findings, and "anxiety," particularly in association with the need to follow small nodules with subsequent scans rather than just "getting them out" [7].

While there is a general call for shared decision-making to help patients determine if they wish to enter a LCS program, the emphasis is on explaining the nature of the risks in a "holistic" way with the patient, at times with the assistance of tools to help the patient make decisions [8]. Some argue that PCPs, who usually know the patient best, should conduct SDM visits and order screening but are hampered by too little time and lack of expertise; others advocate that those associated with the screening program should bear the responsibility [9]. Studies, however, have found that websites associated with screening programs oversell the benefits of screening and rarely mention the risks [10], and recordings of discussions between healthcare providers and patients about LCS rarely mention harms of screening [11].

What is missing from these discussions, although likely implicit in most of them, is the notion of uncertainty. Clinicians generally avoid admitting uncertainty and find it difficult to share with patients that they do not have all the answers [12]. The reality is that much of what we do in medicine has uncertain outcomes and our desire to achieve absolute certainty often carries a tremendous cost, both financial and personal, for the patient. Rather, we should embrace and gain comfort in discussing uncertainty with patients and assist them in the challenge of living with uncertainty [13]. These issues are particularly relevant for three aspects of the discussion with a patient as one embarks on a shared decision-making discussion: the biology of the tumor, the distinction between relative and absolute risk, and the concept of the false positive.

5.2.1 Biology of the Tumor

The entire premise underlying LCS is the notion that primary lung cancers are, on average, relatively slow growing. For a single neoplastic cell to become a visible lesion on a chest radiograph is estimated to take several years. Once a small lesion (<0.8 mm) is detected on CT scan, the likelihood of it spreading within the next year is quite small.

For a patient to be willing to "watch" a lesion for months before the next scan, they must understand that even if the nodule is a cancer (and over 90% of these small nodules are benign), there will be ample time to intervene. Terms like "doubling time" should probably be avoided as one focuses on use of lay language. While we cannot be certain of the biology of any given tumor, can the patient comprehend the notion of a very low probability event and, based on their own psychological make-up, accept this degree of uncertainty? If not, if the thought of a possible tumor growing inside them while they anxiously await the next scan is more than they can bear, then perhaps enrollment in a LCS program is not appropriate for them.

5.2.2 Concept of False Positives

One of the largest sources of morbidity for patients entered into LCS trials is the evaluation and treatment associated with what eventually are found to be benign lesions. Building off of the concept of the biology of the tumor, it is important to discuss with the patient the multiple benign causes of pulmonary nodules. Statistics are often difficult for many patients to fully grasp; the notion that 94% of nodules found in lung cancer screening are not cancer may not resonate with an individual. Inquiring about their understanding of what small and large risk means is important. Describing the nature of the investigations, including surgery, needed to attain certainty and their associated potential complications, will assist the patient in decision-making. There are two levels of uncertainty at this point in the conversation: the uncertainty about whether a particular nodule is cancer, and the uncertainty about experiencing the effects and complications of evaluations to assess any given nodule.

5.2.3 Relative Versus Absolute Risk Reduction

When the NLST trial was published, there was great excitement about the 20% relative reduction in mortality associated with the program [14]. We tend to emphasize relative risk reduction when we think about populations. With lung cancer as the leading cause of cancer death in the United States and around the world, this is an appropriate lens when making decisions for the healthcare of a nation. A given patient, however, is interested, appropriately, in their own health or, in this case, their own risk of dying from lung cancer. With this lens, the benefits of lung cancer screening were much more modest; the mortality fell from 3.3 deaths per 1000 person-years to 2.5 deaths per 1000 person-years.

Efforts have been made to develop increasingly sophisticated risk models and clearly the range of absolute risk may vary considerably among patients being considered for screening [15]. The challenge is to transmit the uncertainty of possible death from lung cancer in a way that addresses the patient's personal circumstances and provides the appropriate data to enable the individual to comprehend the risk in the context of their own situation; 20% reduction of a 10% risk may "feel" much different to the patient than 20% of a 3% risk.

5.2.4 Addressing Uncertainty in Lung Cancer Screening

Clinicians commonly assess a patient's tolerance for pain and discomfort, their willingness to adhere to medication regimens that require taking drugs twice a day versus four times a day, and their fears and anxieties. However, we engage less often in assessing an individual's tolerance for uncertainty. The patient information decision aids developed by the American Thoracic Society provide a wonderful summary of facts about lung cancer and screening yet do not mention the term uncertainty [16]. There are many approaches to shared decision-making [17, 18] but all require including the following key components: introducing choice, describing options, and helping patients explore preferences in a manner that includes confronting risks and the associated uncertainty of outcomes [18].

There are no well-established best strategies for approaching uncertainty with a patient but there is a growing consensus that this should be a part of shared decision-making [19]. As with many aspects of building trust with patients, one should demonstrate sincere curiosity about a patient's views of life, the range of choices and decisions they face on a daily basis, and what they value and fear about their present and future existence. Since the two aspects of uncertainty—aleatoric, defined as uncertainty due to chance, and epistemic, defined as uncertainty due to limited or imperfect knowledge [19]—are both relevant to the patient considering entering lung cancer screening, it is important to have a sense of how the patient views the role of random events in life and their comfort with making decisions with limited knowledge. It may be helpful for providers to convey that uncertainty is inherent in most of what we do in medicine; this is not unusual.

We make decisions based on knowledge, personal values, and what is most important to us as we live our lives. Addressing uncertainty explicitly with patients considering entering a lung cancer screening program is critical not only for the initial decision, but also for the willingness of the patient to undergo baseline and follow-up serial LDCT imaging [20]. We can and must do better.

5.3 Smoking Cessation

The 2020 US Surgeon General's Report was the first one of the series that began in 1964 devoted entirely to smoking cessation. In the Report, surgery, hospitalization, and lung cancer screening were termed "life events" that can trigger smoking cessation attempts, foster uptake of smoking cessation services, and ultimately lead to smoking cessation [21]. The Report concludes that the evidence is "suggestive that fully and consistently integrating standardized, evidence-based smoking cessation interventions into lung cancer screening increases smoking cessation while avoiding potential adverse effects of this screening on cessation outcomes." Consequently, the Center for Medicare and Medicaid Services (CMS) mandate for smoking cessation interventions during the screening process presents an opportunity to deliver this life-saving clinical service [22]. For example, smoking cessation conducted as little as 3 weeks prior to surgery for lung cancer can reduce associated morbidity and mortality [23]. Long-term follow-up of patients who stopped smoking after lung cancer diagnosis and subsequent treatment shows decreased lung cancer progression, increased survival time, and both lower cancer and all-cause mortality compared with those who continue to smoke [24].

5.3.1 Evidence-Based Tobacco Treatment

All the professional societies that have developed lung cancer screening guidelines agree that lung cancer screening is not a substitute for smoking cessation interventions and that evidence-based tobacco treatment should be a standard of care for anyone who smokes or uses tobacco. Most clinical tobacco cessation guidelines emphasize the "5As" approach:

1. Ask patients their smoking status.
2. Advise those who smoke to quit.
3. Assess their willingness to make a quit attempt.
4. Assist in making a quit plan which may include counseling and medication for cessation.
5. Arrange follow-up for those making a quit plan.

Among others, the US Preventive Services Task Force, the American Academy of Family Physicians, the National Comprehensive Cancer Network, the American

Thoracic Society, and the American Society of Clinical Oncology agree that smoking cessation counseling is an essential part of LCS. Many of these groups have also created a variety of professional education materials and programs about cessation. The Association for Treatment of Tobacco Use and Dependence (ATTUD) and the Society for Research on Nicotine and Tobacco jointly issued a guideline in 2016 specifically for smoking cessation in the context of lung cancer screening that summarizes the evidence and suggests treatment strategies for patients who qualify for lung cancer screening. They too found the 5As approach important in this population [25].

There are multiple opportunities during the lung cancer screening process that could potentially increase delivery of tobacco cessation advice, counseling, and treatment. Clinical protocols can be integrated into lung cancer screening to facilitate tobacco cessation services by the PCP or referring provider, screening provider, patient navigator, or other professionals trained to deliver tobacco treatment. The electronic health record (EHR) should be used for documentation and measurement of current and former smoking status, pack-years and time since quitting; templates for smoking cessation should be readily accessible. However, there are deficiencies and limitations in many EHR systems regarding smoking cessation. Greater attention to templates and prompts is needed to improve documentation, accurately assess the smoking pack-year history, identify patients who are eligible for screening, and remind healthcare providers to discuss lung cancer screening and deliver tobacco treatment services. In many healthcare systems, the EHR could be used to integrate smoking cessation service delivery with lung cancer screening care, but this is not always accomplished [26, 27].

Provision of self-help materials (www.smokefree.gov) and referral to community-based programs should be used as part of comprehensive tobacco treatment services that include appropriate follow-up including behavioral counseling and pharmacotherapy. Patients can be referred to quitlines that provide free tobacco counseling, available in all 50 states at the toll-free telephone number 800-QUIT-NOW. Barriers to providing cessation services include time pressures, patient resistance to cessation advice and treatment, inadequate staff training, and lack of reimbursement [28].

5.3.2 Tobacco Therapy and the Shared Decision

The CMS requirement for an initial SDM visit during LCS [22] is intended to help patients understand the potential benefits and harms of LCS; the SDM visit affords an opportunity to discuss smoking cessation as well. Recent studies show, however, that this visit is not easy to adapt to smoking cessation.

Kathuria and colleagues [29] conducted a series of interviews and focus groups to investigate how both physicians and patients view LCS as a "teachable moment" for smoking cessation discussions; the results provide a mixed picture. Physicians often saw the smoking cessation intervention as distinct from SDM with little connection between the two. Most physicians believed that receipt of LCS results would affect patient motivation; however, not all thought it would be a "wake-up call" to stop smoking. For many patients, the LCS process encouraged them to rethink their smoking behavior and consider cessation. Cessation discussions did not consistently occur from the viewpoint of either physicians or patients, and the authors concluded that there were many missed opportunities for cessation counseling.

Golden et al. [30], in a set of in-depth interviews, came to similar conclusions about LCS and smoking cessation discussions between patients and physicians. In a retrospective study of SDM practices, Shen et al. [31] found that 39% of patients received at least one smoking cessation resource, and only 5% received both counseling and pharmacotherapy for cessation. Patients in this study were more likely to receive smoking cessation advice from their PCP or specialist, as opposed to others within the screening process.

There are scant data about how to incorporate smoking cessation into the radiology encounter for low-dose chest CT. While the American College of Radiology offers resources such as archived webinars and presentations about smoking cessation on its website, it is unclear how deeply these materials have penetrated into practice. Staff who conduct the screening CT scan are not likely to have had formal training about smoking cessation and its role in LCS, have time constraints, and may not consider this to be part of their job [32].

More research is needed to determine how best to include smoking cessation into the radiology encounter in LCS settings.

5.3.3   Personalized Risk Assessment to Support Quitting

Discussions about LCS results might occur with specialist physicians or the patient's PCP. Regardless of the venue or the screening results, an opportunity exists to discuss the importance of smoking cessation by integrating smoking cessation counseling during the post-screening period and incorporating cessation advice into discussions of scan results. This approach is a way to personalize risk assessments to motivate and support smoking cessation. Many patients in the Kathuria focus groups reported that this was the most powerful time in the LCS process to encourage cessation [29]. In some studies (but not all), abnormal findings on LCS predicted subsequent smoking cessation [33]. A study comparing patients referred versus those not referred for evaluation of screening abnormalities found increased rates of smoking cessation at 1 year among referred patients [34].

Annual follow-up LDCT scans are recommended for eligible persons, providing an opportunity for smoking cessation advice, counseling, and treatment. It is important to repeat the assessment of smoking status and inquire about any interval health issues to personalize quitting advice. Park et al. [28] surveyed PCPs who took part in the National Lung Screening Trial to explore delivery of "5As" tobacco cessation services after LCS, and smoking behavior changes among screened patients.

Delivery of the elements of the 5As 1 year after screening were: ask, 77.2%; advise, 75.6%; assess, 63.4%; assist, 56.4%; and arrange follow-up, 10.4%. Only the "assist" and "arrange" activities were associated with significant smoking cessation behavior among patients (40% and 46% increase in the odds of quitting, respectively), indicating that more active contact between the patient and physician at LCS follow-up resulted in better cessation outcomes.

5.3.4 Barriers to Quitting

Patients who undergo LCS have a wide range of beliefs, fears, and concerns about screening that may influence their uptake of tobacco cessation advice [35, 36]. Some patients in screening programs who smoke have little interest in quitting [37, 38], but others may be focused on health issues such as COPD or another smoking-related disease and accept cessation advice more readily. Several patient characteristics are associated with difficulty in quitting smoking, including higher nicotine dependence, heavier smoking intensity, longer smoking duration, being single, lower education, and second-hand smoke exposure in the home [33, 39]. It is important to address fatalism and nihilism among these higher-risk, older patients and emphasize the evidence for the benefits of cessation among older persons who smoke such as improving fatigue and dyspnea, as well as reducing the risk of death from lung cancer and other tobacco-related diseases [40, 41].

There are also provider and systems-level barriers to incorporating tobacco treatment into LCS. A survey of LCS site coordinators in the USA found that the health system placed a high priority on promoting smoking cessation among lung cancer screening enrollees; patients were routinely asked about their current smoking status (98.9%) and current smokers were regularly advised to quit (91.4%). Fewer sites, however, provided cessation counseling (57%) or referred smokers to a quitline (60.2%) and a minority (36.6%) routinely recommended cessation medications [42]. Barriers to cessation treatment included time pressure, perceived poor patient motivation for and resistance to cessation advice and treatment, inadequate staff training, and reimbursement issues [42, 43].

Inadequate training and lack of options for referral to a professional with expertise in tobacco treatment is frequently cited as a barrier for integration of cessation services in LCS. Brief physician training has been shown to increase delivery of evidence-based tobacco treatment [44, 45]. However, going beyond the 5As and delivering in-depth counseling and pharmacotherapy requires more intensive training. Since 2004 intensive tobacco treatment training programs, 22 of which are accredited by the Council for Tobacco Treatment Training Programs, have conducted nationwide training of Certified Tobacco Treatment Specialists (CTTS). Given the problems with inadequate tobacco cessation education in LCS programs, Roughgarden et al. [46] recently called for more use of tobacco treatment specialists by LCS sites to increase delivery of evidence-based smoking cessation services.

Finally, researchers point to the paucity of good data on smoking cessation in the setting of LCS and have called for further research on a variety of issues including cessation elements, format, timing, setting, and patient risk perception on motivation and success in stopping smoking [24, 42, 47–49]. Most clinical trials related to tobacco cessation have not incorporated the unique issues regarding persons who are eligible for LCS and the systems that have been created to implement screening. The SCALE (Smoking Cessation within the Context of Lung Cancer Screening) collaboration is currently developing protocols to study a wide range of issues to improve tobacco cessation interventions in LCS settings [50].

5.4 Innovation in Lung Screening and Decision Support Tools

5.4.1 What Is Innovation?

The most successful innovations begin by asking the end user what they want. In the case of lung screening, it starts with asking eligible patients what a good decision aid might look like. Does the individual prefer written material that reviews false positives and false negatives and discusses the risk/benefit ratio in percentages, or might they prefer an experiential tool designed to engage patients in a way that allows them to pause and consider risk and benefits while also encouraging individuals 50–80 years old to consider their overall lung health, and the behaviors they might modify to achieve the quality of life they imagine and hope for as they approach the last quarter of life? Of course, the solution does not demand an "either/or" choice, and different individuals may respond more or less to a particular intervention.

5.4.2 Current Educational Tools Are Lacking

Medical information is often abstract and complex for patients and their loved ones as they struggle to understand what is happening within their own bodies. Patients forget up to 80% of the information presented to them almost immediately after their clinical consultations [51–53], with up to 50% of the information retained being remembered inaccurately [53, 54]. This poor understanding can adversely affect patient anxiety [55], compliance [56, 57], provider trust [58], satisfaction [59], shared medical decision-making [60, 61], and clinical outcomes [62–64]. Having a family member, friend, or support person accompany them to crucial appointments to listen and take notes while the patient does their best to process what they are hearing can be particularly helpful in supporting recall. One of the core challenges in patient education is to effectively communicate unfamiliar and complicated medical information or concepts to patients in a format they can easily understand.

These communication issues are likely compounded by providers' own bias of overestimating how well they teach and incorrectly perceiving patients understand more than they actually do [65–67]. Moreover, providers often struggle to understand the experience of being the patient [68, 69], which can reduce their ability to relate to and show empathy for the patient [70]. In terms of patient education approaches, studies have shown that a "verbal discussion" when used alone is the least effective educational tool and should be combined with other methods [71–73].

5.4.3   Experiential Learning and Understanding Pulmonary Nodules

It is important to pause and consider whether the instruments currently in use are designed to enhance process measures but may not be relevant to patients. Decision aids that tend to focus on knowledge may do nothing to reduce the distress a patient may feel when asked to consider undergoing LCS by their PCP or is considering self-referral [74]. If SDM is intended to engage patients in a way that is meaningful to each unique patient, what might the lung screening shared decision-making conversation include to enhance the patient experience?

Despite the low risk of malignancy, several studies indicate that lung nodule findings lead to clinically significant distress in as many as 25% of patients [75]. Patients often find the term "nodule" mystifying but intuitively feel it may somehow increase the risk of lung cancer [76]. These patients tend to overestimate their risk of lung cancer which may be the consequence of the observation that patients often receive inadequate information about their nodule and want more information about the risk their nodule poses for them [77].

To improve patient understanding of the risk posed by one or more pulmonary nodules on CT chest scans, Maine Health, Maine Cancer Care Network, and The Department of Thoracic Oncology supported the development and clinical investigation of a 3D Printed Lung Nodule Tool to explore whether it would help providers educate patients about lung nodules during a SDM consult.

The lung nodule patient education tool (Fig. 5.1) was piloted during shared decision-making consults to explain the significance of nodule size, appearance, and malignancy risk.

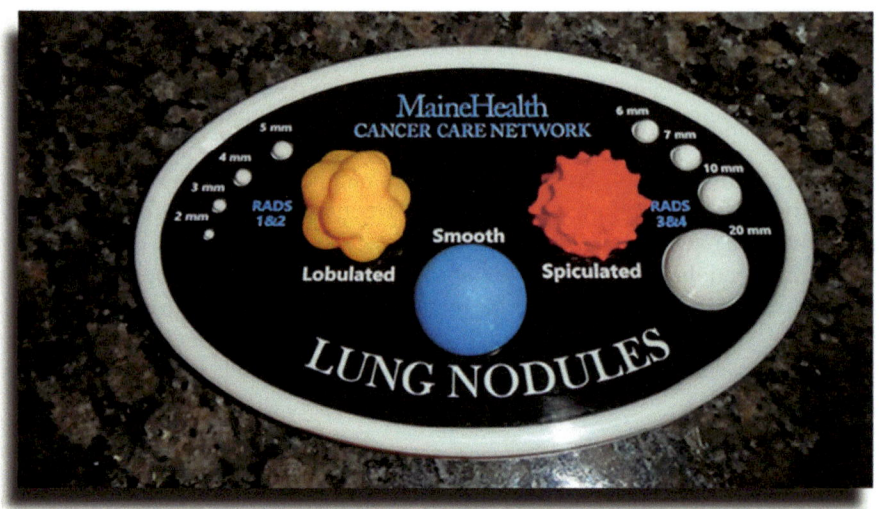

Fig. 5.1 3D Lung nodule education tool

5.4.4 Measuring the Effectiveness of a Tactile Lung Nodule Tool

Effectiveness of the tool was assessed through a brief patient survey, which was completed by 31 patients. Preliminary data revealed patients found the 3D lung nodule tool helpful with improved overall understanding of lung nodules in terms of nodule size, appearance, and significance. The average score for helpfulness (1 being not helpful and 10 being extremely helpful) was 9.4 out of 10 (Fig. 5.2). The initial data demonstrated that use of a patient education lung nodule tool during lung screening shared decision-making supported patient understanding of nodules, improved communication, and reduced patient anxiety.

The lung nodule tool proved to be particularly helpful during the pandemic when telehealth consults became an essential platform in delivering patient care. The tool could be held to the camera during a patient telehealth consult, which gave patients an opportunity to engage visually with the tool and further supported their understanding of pulmonary nodule sizing in contrast to metric numerical values to characterize nodule size.

This technique provided a unique opportunity to reach rural patients allowing them to undergo LDCT imaging closer to home rather than driving 1–2 h to have a SDM consult with a provider prior to imaging.

on a scale from 1 (*not helpful*) to 10 (exremely)
not helpful), please rate the 3D lung nodule tool.

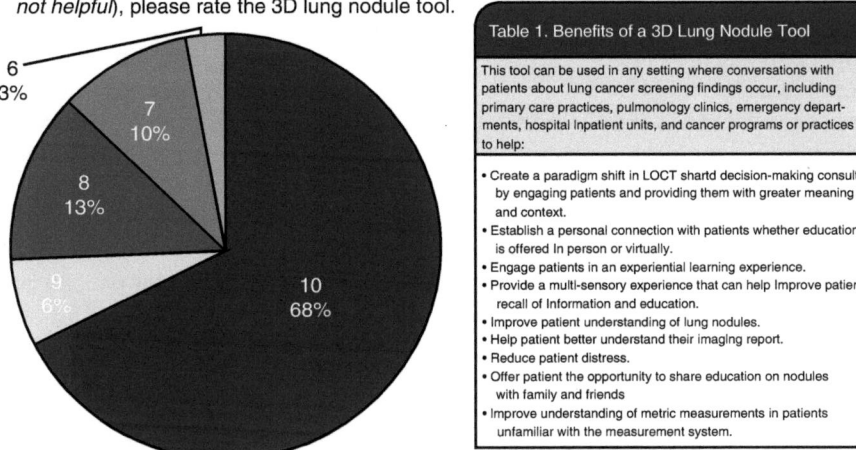

Table 1. Benefits of a 3D Lung Nodule Tool

This tool can be used in any setting where conversations with patients about lung cancer screening findings occur, including primary care practices, pulmonology clinics, emergency departments, hospital inpatient units, and cancer programs or practices to help:

• Create a paradigm shift in LOCT shartd decision-making consults by engaging patients and providing them with greater meaning and context.
• Establish a personal connection with patients whether education is offered In person or virtually.
• Engage patients in an experiential learning experience.
• Provide a multi-sensory experience that can help Improve patient recall of Information and education.
• Improve patient understanding of lung nodules.
• Help patient better understand their imaging report.
• Reduce patient distress.
• Offer patient the opportunity to share education on nodules with family and friends
• Improve understanding of metric measurements in patients unfamiliar with the measurement system.

LDCT = low-dose computed tomography.

Fig. 5.2 Benefits of a lung nodule tool to reduce anxiety through knowledge

5.4.5 *Innovations for Rural Engagement and Supporting Quitting*

During the SDM discussion, patients frequently ask "Is there anything else that can help me quit smoking? I've tried everything." Currently, a cell phone app called "The Tobacco Leaf App" is under development. Designed to support patients who want to quit smoking within the context of lung screening, the app tracks monetary gain or loss by smoking, life months and years lost or gained by continuing/discontinuing smoking, pulmonary nodule size and location tracking, emphysema extent and location, recommended follow-up, and reminders for the patient about their next LDCT scan.

The option of providing a SDM video on an organizational website is currently being adapted by lung screening sites across the country. Such a video may offer content typically discussed with a provider during a LCS shared decision-making consult, and has the ability to offer information about incidental findings often found on LDCT imaging such as emphysema and atherosclerosis. It also offers remote rural patients, for whom traveling long distances to see a doctor may be a major impediment to care, an opportunity to understand lung screening and make a decision that is right for them. This format proved particularly useful and received emergency use authorization for use during the SARS-COV 2 pandemic.

5.4.6   Virtual Reality: Next Generational Teaching Tool

In the goal of shared medical decision-making with patients, being fully informed is a prerequisite. Additional tools may be needed to effectively communicate with patients to allow them to truly understand what is happening within their own bodies.

One newer approach is the use of virtual reality (VR). Patients' own medical imaging is personalized and often contains a tremendous amount of information about their possible disease and its relationship with adjacent structures and organs, information critical to provide important context in medical discussions. However, the current 2D planar medical imaging format is often unfamiliar for patients and has been considered equivalent to looking at a Rorschach inkblot. Using VR, these individual data image slices can be presented in their entirety in a 3D volume, allowing patients to intuitively see and directly interact with 3D representations of themselves. VR is supported as an educational tool by multiple learning theories including embodiment [78], situational [79], and constructivist learning [80] in that a patient is not just hearing or seeing but experiencing their information. Additionally, presenting 3D information in 3D versus 2D format can lower cognitive load which is important for improved learning [81]. More recently, the FDA is now recognizing medical extended reality in medicine. Although there are limited studies using VR to inform patients, they have resulted in higher satisfaction, increased engagement and overwhelming preference for VR in clinical consultations [82–86]. Holt et al. conducted a prospective quantitative and qualitative study for cancer patients and their loved ones using VR. Research is underway utilizing VR to show patients the medical imaging of their tumors and radiation treatment in 3D (Fig. 5.3) [87]. Within the study, 25 separate VR sessions were conducted from patient ages of 11–95 years old with a median time of 5 months from the time of their diagnosis to

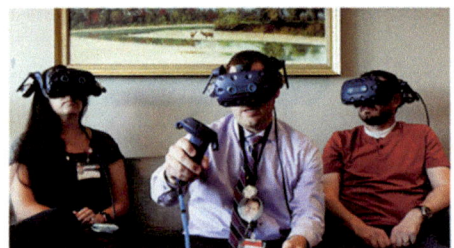

University of Colorado Cancer Center, UCHealth-Oncology Services
Aurora, Colorado

3D Virtual Reality: Changing the Standard of Care for Patients with Cancer and Their Caregivers

Douglas Holt, MD, Chief Resident, Radiation Oncology

Virtual reality (VR) is uniquely positioned to improve patient understanding of cancer and its treatments. During clinical consultations, radiation oncology staff use a mobile VR cart to provide 3D patient-specific CT, MRI, and PET-CT imaging to enhance provider and patient interaction, improve patient education, and reduce patient distress. Hear results from a clinical study that captured both quantitative and qualitative data on patient acceptance and perceived usefulness of VR in cancer education and treatment.

Fig. 5.3 Improving patient understanding through virtual reality

the VR imaging review [87]. Patients and their caregivers reported VR increased their understanding of their disease from a mean of 5.6 (pre-VR) to 9.2 (post-VR; 0 = no understanding, 10 = full understanding) in a 5–7-min session [87]. Ninety-seven percent preferred VR over standard 2D computer imaging review [87]. Additionally, 83% of participants reported VR as the top educational tool over all other standard teaching methods with 97% agreeing that VR should be the standard of care for patients during their clinical consultations [87].

From the qualitative analysis of semi-structured interviews, patients noted VR presented the information in a format that was simple and easy to comprehend [87]. In addition, VR provided additional understanding and allowed improved engagement with providers and their treatment [87]. Interestingly, VR had a positive impact on patients' attitudes towards modifying their behaviors in regard to compliance with recommendations.

This impact on patient behavior, which might be particularly important when advising patients to pursue LCS and smoking cessation, has been demonstrated in other disease states. In a study involving patients with HIV, half of the group experienced an interactive session with VR to visualize white blood cells, seeing the impact of a HIV infection to the cells along with the effect of treatment with HIV antiviral medications [88]. As a result, the group with the VR session had a decrease in their HIV viral load compared to no change in the standard consultation group, indicating improved adherence to their antiviral therapy [88].

These findings along with previous studies warrant further investigation of the use of VR in patient education, including SDM discussions for LCS, image results, and smoking cessation.

Innovations in patient health education are key to a patient's engagement toward good health. By collaborating with patients to educate and design an individualized plan of care, we develop meaningful health goals that mirror the needs of the individual patient while simultaneously encouraging health autonomy.

References

1. Lowenstein LM, Deyter GMR, Nishi S, Wang T, Volk RJ. Shared decision-making conversations and smoking cessation interventions: critical components of low-dose CT lung cancer screening programs. Transl Lung Cancer Res. 2018;7(3):254–71. https://doi.org/10.21037/tlcr.2018.05.10.
2. Hurley V, Rodriguez H, Kearing S, Wang Y, Leung M, Shortell S. The impact of decision aids on adults considering hip or knee surgery. Health Aff (Millwood). 2020;39(1):100–7. https://doi.org/10.1377/hlthaff.2019.00100.
3. Slatore C, Wiener RS. Pulmonary nodules, a small problem for many, severe distress for some, and how to communicate about it. 2018. https://doi.org/10.1016/j.chest2017.10.013.
4. Volk R, Lowenstein L, Leal V, Escoto K, Cantor S, Munden R, et al. Effect of a patient decision aid on lung cancer screening. Decision-making by persons who smoke: a randomized clinical trial. JAMA Netw Open. 2020;3(1):e1920362. https://doi.org/10.1001/jamanetworkopen.2019.20362.

5. Veroff D, Marr A, Wennberg D. Enhanced support for shared decision making reduced costs of care for patients with preference-sensitive conditions. Health Aff (Millwood). 2013;32(2):285–93. https://doi.org/10.1377/hlthaff.2011.0941.
6. National Lung Cancer Screening Trail Writing Team. Reduced lung-cancer mortality with low-dose computed tomographic screening. N Engl J Med. 2011;365:395–409.
7. Smetana GW, Boiselle PM, Schwartzstein RM. Screening for lung cancer with low-dose computed tomography: grand rounds discussion from the Beth Israel Deaconess Medical Center. Ann Intern Med. 2015;162:577–82.
8. Triplette M, Kross EK, Mann BA, Elmore JG, Slatore CG, Shahrir S, Romine PE, Frederick PD, Chorthers K. An assessment of primary care and pulmonary provider perspectives on lung cancer screening. Ann Am Thorac Soc. 2018;15:69–75.
9. Powell CA. Should only primary care physicians provide shared decision-making services to discuss the risks/benefits for a low-dose chest CT scan for lung cancer screening? No Chest. 2016. PMID: 28041887.
10. Clark SD, Reuland DS, Enyioha C, Jonas DE. Assessment of lung cancer screening program websites. JAMA Intern Med. 2020;180:824–30.
11. Brenner AT, Malo TL, Margolis M, Lafata JE, Shynah J, Vu Maihan B, Reuland DS. Evaluating shared decision making for lung cancer screening. JAMA Intern Med. 2018;178:131–6.
12. Simpkin AL, Schwartzstein RM. Tolerating uncertainty—the next medical revolution? N Engl J Med. 2016;375:1713–5.
13. Dunlop M, Schwartzstein RM. Reducing diagnostic error in the intensive care unit: uncertainty when teaching clinical reasoning. ATS Sch. 2020;1:364–71.
14. Jonas DE, Reuland DS, Reddy SM, Nagle M, Clark SD, Weber RP, Enyioha C, Malo TL, Brenner AT, Armstrong C, Coker-Schwimmer M, Middleton JC, Voisin C, Harris RP. Screening for lung cancer with low dose computed tomography: updated evidence report and systematic review for the US Preventive Services Task Force. JAMA. 2021;325:971–87.
15. Toumazis I, Bastani M, Han SS, Plevritis. Risk-based lung cancer screening: a systematic review. Lung Cancer. 2020;147:154–86.
16. ATS patient information. Lung cancer screening: what is screening and what does it have to do with lung cancer? Am J Respir Crit Care Med. 2021;204:19–20.
17. Tanner NT, Silvestri GA. Shared decision-making and lung cancer screening. Chest. 2019;155:21–4.
18. Armstrong KA, Metlay JP. Annals clinical decision-making: communicating risk and engaging patients in shared decision-making. Ann Intern Med. 2020;172(10):688–93.
19. Simpkin AL, Armstrong KA. Communicating uncertainty: a narrative review and framework for future research. J Gen Intern Med. 2019;34:2586–91.
20. Sakoda LC, Henderson LM, Rivera MP. Adherence to lung cancer screening: what exactly are we talking about? Ann Am Thorac Soc. 2021;18:1951–2.
21. U.S. Department of Health and Human Services. Smoking cessation: a report of the surgeon general. Atlanta, GA: U.S. Department of Health and Human Services, Centers for Disease Control and Prevention, National Center for Chronic Disease Prevention and Health Promotion, Office on Smoking and Health; 2020.
22. Centers for Medicare & Medicaid Services. NCA—screening for lung cancer with low dose cOMPUTED TOMOGRaphy (LDCT) (CAG-00439R)—proposed decision memo November 17, 2021. https://www.cms.gov/medicare-coverage-database/view/ncacal-decision-memo.aspx?proposed=Y&ncaid=304&. Accessed 6 Dec 2021.
23. Heiden BT, Eaton DB Jr, Chang SH, et al. Assessment of duration of smoking cessation prior to surgical treatment of non-small cell lung cancer. Ann Surg 2021. https://doi.org/10.1097/SLA.0000000000005312. Epub ahead of print.
24. Sheikh M, Mukeriya A, Shangina O, et al. Postdiagnosis smoking cessation and reduced risk for lung cancer progression and mortality : a prospective cohort study. Ann Intern Med. 2021;174(9):1232–9.
25. Fucito LM, Czabafy S, Hendricks PS, et al. Pairing smoking-cessation services with lung cancer screening: a clinical guideline from the association for the treatment of tobacco use and dependence and the Society for Research on Nicotine and Tobacco. Cancer. 2016;122(8):1150–9.

26. Jose T, Hays JT, Warner DO. Improved documentation of electronic cigarette use in an electronic health record. Int J Environ Res Public Health. 2020;17(16):5908.
27. Peterson E, Harris K, Farjah F, et al. Improving smoking history documentation in the electronic health record for lung cancer risk assessment and screening in primary care: a case study. Healthc (Amst). 2021;9(4):100578.
28. Park ER, Gareen IF, Japuntich S, et al. Primary care provider-delivered smoking cessation interventions and smoking cessation among participants in the National Lung Screening Trial. JAMA Intern Med. 2015;175(9):1509–16.
29. Kathuria H, Koppelman E, Borrelli B, et al. Patient-physician discussions on lung cancer screening: a missed teachable moment to promote smoking cessation. Nicotine Tob Res. 2020;22(3):431–9.
30. Golden SE, Ono SS, Melzer A, et al. "I already know that smoking ain't good for me": patient and clinician perspectives on lung cancer screening decision-making discussions as a teachable moment. Chest. 2020;158(3):1250–9.
31. Shen J, Crothers K, Kross EK, et al. Provision of smoking cessation resources in the context of in-person shared decision-making for lung cancer screening. Chest. 2021;160(2):765–75.
32. Aberle DR. Implementing lung cancer screening: the US experience. Clin Radiol. 2017;72(5):401–6.
33. Tammemägi MC, Berg CD, Riley TL, et al. Impact of lung cancer screening results on smoking cessation. J Natl Cancer Inst. 2014;106(6):dju084.
34. Styn MA, Land SR, Perkins KA, et al. Smoking behavior 1 year after computed tomography screening for lung cancer: effect of physician referral for abnormal CT findings. Cancer Epidemiol Biomark Prev. 2009;18(12):3484–9.
35. Brain K, Carter B, Lifford KJ, et al. Impact of low-dose CT screening on smoking cessation among high-risk participants in the UK Lung Cancer Screening Trial. Thorax. 2017;72(10):912–8.
36. Fagerlin A, Sepucha KR, Couper MP, et al. Patients' knowledge about 9 common health conditions: the DECISIONS survey. Med Decis Mak. 2010;30(5 Suppl):35S–52S.
37. Clark MA, Gorelick JJ, Sicks JD, et al. The relations between false positive and negative screens and smoking cessation and relapse in the National Lung Screening Trial: implications for public health. Nicotine Tob Res. 2016;18(1):17–24.
38. Taylor KL, Cox LS, Zincke N, Mehta L, McGuire C, Gelmann E. Lung cancer screening as a teachable moment for smoking cessation. Lung Cancer. 2007;56(1):125–34.
39. Rojewski AM, Tanner NT, Dai L, et al. Tobacco dependence predicts higher lung cancer and mortality rates and lower rates of smoking cessation in the National Lung Screening Trial. Chest. 2018;154(1):110–8.
40. Gellert C, Schottker B, Brenner H. Smoking and all-cause mortality in older people: systematic review and meta-analysis. Arch Intern Med. 2012;172(11):837–44.
41. Woloshin S, Schwartz LM, Welch HG. The risk of death by age, sex, and smoking status in the United States: putting health risks in context. J Natl Cancer Inst. 2008;100(12):845–53.
42. Ostroff JS, Copeland A, Borderud SP, et al. Readiness of lung cancer screening sites to deliver smoking cessation treatment: current practices, organizational priority, and perceived barriers. Nicotine Tob Res. 2016;18(5):1067–75.
43. Melzer AC, Golden SE, Ono SS, et al. "We just never have enough time": clinician views of lung cancer screening processes and implementation. Ann Am Thorac Soc. 2020. https://doi.org/10.1513/AnnalsATS.202003-262OC. Epub ahead of print.
44. Bauer A, Brenner L, Moser J, et al. The effects of a short-term physician training on smoking cessation in a university pulmonary department. Ger Med Sci. 2020;18:Doc06.
45. Kastaun S, Leve V, Hildebrandt J, et al. Training general practitioners in the ABC versus 5As method of delivering stop-smoking advice: a pragmatic, two-arm cluster randomised controlled trial. ERJ Open Res. 2021;7(3):00621-2020.
46. Roughgarden KL, Toll BA, Tanner NT, et al. Tobacco treatment specialist training for lung cancer screening providers. Am J Prev Med. 2021;61(5):765–8.

47. Minnix JA, Karam-Hage M, Blalock JA, et al. The importance of incorporating smoking cessation into lung cancer screening. Transl Lung Cancer Res. 2018;7(3):272–80.
48. Iaccarino JM, Duran C, Slatore CG, et al. Combining smoking cessation interventions with LDCT lung cancer screening: a systematic review. Prev Med. 2019;121:24–32.
49. Kathuria H, Detterbeck FC, Fathi JT, et al. ATS assembly on thoracic oncology. Stakeholder research priorities for smoking cessation interventions within lung cancer screening programs. An official American Thoracic Society research statement. Am J Respir Crit Care Med. 2017;196(9):1202–12.
50. Joseph AM, Rothman AJ, Almirall D, et al. Lung cancer screening and smoking cessation clinical trials. SCALE (smoking cessation within the context of lung cancer screening) Collaboration. Am J Respir Crit Care Med. 2018;197(2):172–82.
51. McGuire LC. Remembering what the doctor said: organization and adults' memory for medical information. Exp Aging Res. 1996;22(4):403–28. https://doi.org/10.1080/03610739608254020.
52. Laws MB, Lee Y, Taubin T, Rogers WH, Wilson IB. Factors associated with patient recall of key information in ambulatory specialty care visits: results of an innovative methodology. PLoS One. 2018;13(2):e0191940. https://doi.org/10.1371/journal.pone.0191940.
53. Kessels RP. Patients' memory for medical information. J R Soc Med. 2003;96(5):219–22. https://doi.org/10.1258/jrsm.96.5.219.
54. Anderson JL, Dodman S, Kopelman M, Fleming A. Patient information recall in a rheumatology clinic. Rheumatol Rehabil. 1979;18(1):18–22. https://doi.org/10.1093/rheumatology/18.1.18.
55. Fernsler JI, Cannon CA. The whys of patient education. Semin Oncol Nurs. 1991;7(2):79–86. https://doi.org/10.1016/0749-2081(91)90085-4.
56. Gold DT, McClung B. Approaches to patient education: emphasizing the long-term value of compliance and persistence. Am J Med. 2006;119(4 Suppl 1):S32–7. https://doi.org/10.1016/j.amjmed.2005.12.021.
57. Sundaresan P, King M, Stockler M, Costa D, Milross C. Barriers to radiotherapy utilization: consumer perceptions of issues influencing radiotherapy-related decisions. Asia Pac J Clin Oncol. 2017;13(5):e489–96. https://doi.org/10.1111/ajco.12579.
58. Grant SB. Are there blueprints for building a strong patient-physician relationship? Virtual Mentor. 2009;11(3):232–6. https://doi.org/10.1001/virtualmentor.2009.11.3.jdsc1-0903.
59. Press Ganey: public reporting gives huge boost to patient satisfaction. Healthcare Benchmarks Qual Improv. 2008;15(12):121–3.
60. Hess CB, Chen AM. Measuring psychosocial functioning in the radiation oncology clinic: a systematic review. Psychooncology. 2014;23(8):841–54. https://doi.org/10.1002/pon.3521.
61. Takahashi T, Hondo M, Nishimura K, et al. Evaluation of quality of life and psychological response in cancer patients treated with radiotherapy. Radiat Med. 2008;26(7):396–401. https://doi.org/10.1007/s11604-008-0248-5.
62. Martin LR, Williams SL, Haskard KB, Dimatteo MR. The challenge of patient adherence. Ther Clin Risk Manag. 2005;1(3):189–99.
63. Buetow S. The scope for the involvement of patients in their consultations with health professionals: rights, responsibilities and preferences of patients. J Med Ethics. 1998;24(4):243–7. https://doi.org/10.1136/jme.24.4.243.
64. Chipidza FE, Wallwork RS, Stern TA. Impact of the doctor-patient relationship. Prim Care Companion CNS Disord. 2015;17(5). https://doi.org/10.4088/PCC.15f01840.
65. Stewart MA. Effective physician-patient communication and health outcomes: a review. CMAJ. 1995;152(9):1423–33.
66. Tongue JR, Epps HR, Forese LL. Communication skills. Instr Course Lect. 2005;54:3–9.
67. Jukic M, Kozina S, Kardum G, Hogg R, Kvolik S. Physicians overestimate patient's knowledge of the process of informed consent: a cross-sectional study. Med Glas (Zenica). 2011;8(1):39–45.
68. Norden C. I had to get cancer to become a more empathetic doctor. Ann Intern Med. 2016;165(7):525–6. https://doi.org/10.7326/M16-1243.

69. Kemp J, Zars C. A tale of two perspectives on cancer: what I wish I knew before cancer—radiologist and patient perspectives. J Am Coll Radiol. 2016;13(12):1625–7.
70. Wiemann C. The "curse of knowledge," or why intuition about teaching often fails. APS News. 2007;16(10).
71. Johnson A, Sandford J. Written and verbal information versus verbal information only for patients being discharged from acute hospital settings to home: systematic review. Health Educ Res. 2005;20(4):423–9.
72. Theis SL, Johnson JH. Strategies for teaching patients: a meta-analysis. Clin Nurse Spec. 1995;9(2):100–5, 120.
73. Friedman AJ, Cosby R, Boyko S, Hatton-Bauer J, Turnbull G. Effective teaching strategies and methods of delivery for patient education: a systematic review and practice guideline recommendations. J Cancer Educ. 2011;26(1):12–21.
74. Slatore C, Soylemez R. Wiener pulmonary nodules, a small problem for many, severe distress for some, and how to communicate about it. Chest. 2018;153(4):1004–15. https://doi.org/10.1016/j.chest2017.10.013.
75. Roelke T. 3D lung nodule tool fills a gap in patient care, reducing distress and improving shared decision making. Oncol Issues. 2021;36(2).
76. Slatore C, Press N, Au D, Curtis R, Wiener R. What the heck is a "nodule"? A qualitative study of veteran's with pulmonary nodules. Ann Am Thorac Soc. 2013;10(4):330–5.
77. Golden S, Wiener R, Sullivan D, Ganzini L, Slatore C. Primary care providers and a system problem. A qualitative study of clinicians caring for patients with incidental pulmonary nodules. Chest. 2015;148(6):1422–9.
78. Wilson M. Six views of embodied cognition. Psychon Bull Rev. 2002;9(4):625–36.
79. Lave J, Wenger E. Situated learning: legitimate peripheral participation. Cambridge: Cambridge University Press; 1991.
80. Fokides E, Tsolakidis C. Virtual reality in education: a theoretical approach for road safety training to students. Eur J Open Distance E-learning. 2008;11(2)
81. Dan A, Reiner M. EEG-based cognitive load of processing events in 3D virtual worlds is lower than processing events in 2D displays. Int J Psychophysiol. 2017;122:75–84.
82. Pandrangi VC, Gaston B, Appelbaum NP, Albuquerque FC Jr, Levy MM, Larson RA. The application of virtual reality in patient education. Ann Vasc Surg. 2019;59:184–9. https://doi.org/10.1016/j.avsg.2019.01.015.
83. Collins MK, Ding VY, Ball RL, Dolce DL, Henderson JM, Halpern CH. Novel application of virtual reality in patient engagement for deep brain stimulation: a pilot study. Brain Stimul. 2018;11(4):935–7.
84. House PM, Pelzl S, Furrer S, et al. Use of the mixed reality tool "VSI patient education" for more comprehensible and imaginable patient educations before epilepsy surgery and stereotactic implantation of DBS or stereo-EEG electrodes. Epilepsy Res. 2020;159:106247.
85. Louis R, Cagigas J, Brant-Zawadzki M, Ricks M. Impact of neurosurgical consultation with 360-degree virtual reality technology on patient engagement and satisfaction. Neurosurg Open. 2020;1(3):1–9.
86. Castellanos JM, Yefimov A, Dang PN. 360-degree virtual reality consultation for the structural heart disease patient. Struct Heart. 2020;4(3):230–5.
87. Holt D, Carr A, Roberts S, et al. 3D virtual reality volumetric imaging review in cancer patients' understanding and education of their disease and treatment. Int J Radiat Oncol Biol Phys. 2021;111(3):e157.
88. Liran O, Dasher R, Kaeochinda K. Using virtual reality to improve antiretroviral therapy adherence in the treatment of HIV: open-label repeated measure study. Interact J Med Res. 2019;8(2):e13698. https://doi.org/10.2196/13698.

Chapter 6
Lung Cancer Screening Results and Tracking

Debra S. Dyer and Kim L. Sandler

6.1 Ordering a LCS CT

An order is required for a LCS CT to be performed. The order can be written or electronic. An order is needed for the initial baseline low-dose CT (LDCT) and for the subsequent annual LDCTs.

The order must be placed by a Licensed Independent Practitioner (LIP). The National Provider Identifier (NPI) number of the ordering provider must be supplied.

The patient eligibility criteria for LCS as recommended by the USPSTF [1] are:

Age 50–80 years
Current tobacco use or quit smoking within the past 15 years
At least 20 pack-year history of smoking
Asymptomatic (no signs or symptoms of lung cancer)

The order needs to document the eligibility criteria including the patient's date-of-birth, actual pack-year history of tobacco use, and whether the patient is currently smoking or if previously smoked, the years since quit. The order must include a statement that the patient is asymptomatic with no signs or symptoms of lung cancer such as unexplained weight loss or hemoptysis. For Medicare beneficiaries, the order must also include documentation that the patient has participated in a Shared Decision Making (SDM) visit with a licensed provider [2]. For the patient who currently smokes, Medicare also requires documentation that the patient

D. S. Dyer (✉)
Department of Radiology, National Jewish Health, Denver, CO, USA
e-mail: DyerD@NJHealth.org

K. L. Sandler
Department of Radiology and Radiological Sciences, Vanderbilt University Medical Center, Nashville, TN, USA

© The Author(s), under exclusive license to Springer Nature Switzerland AG 2022
J. V. Baptiste et al. (eds.), *Lung Cancer Screening*,
https://doi.org/10.1007/978-3-031-10662-0_6

105

received counseling on tobacco cessation and was offered a referral to smoking cessation services.

The appropriate ICD-10 diagnosis codes must be included in the order. Code F17.21 is utilized for persons who currently smoke (nicotine dependence) and code Z87.891 is used for persons who have previously smoked (personal history of nicotine dependence).

In a decentralized LCS Program, the order is typically submitted by the primary care provider (PCP) or other licensed ordering provider. In a centralized LCS program, the order and SDM visit are usually placed by clinical providers associated with the LCS program. The program helps manage the care continuum for the patient following the LDCT.

Some individuals may be deemed appropriate for LCS through risk-prediction models such as the Prostate, Lung, Colorectal and Ovarian (PLCO) M2012 model. Such models incorporate demographic and clinical factors and have been found to be more sensitive for lung cancer detection than the age and smoking criteria based on the NLST [3, 4]. The use of a risk assessment model has also been shown to help address health disparities in LCS [5]. Other advanced risk assessment models include the Bach model, the Lung Cancer Risk Assessment Tool (LCRAT), and the Lung Cancer Death Risk Assessment (LCDRAT). Typically, a risk of 1.5% or greater is considered "high risk" for lung cancer [4]. Since most insurers do not reimburse for LCS CT based on these criteria, individuals would need to have their CTs done on a self-pay basis. In this situation, the order should include the risk model used, the data points used to determine the risk status and the calculated risk.

It is important the order indicate if a patient has had a prior chest CT that can be used for comparison. The location and approximate date of the prior exam should be provided. Comparison exams are especially important for patients having an initial baseline LCS CT. Any interval diagnostic chest CTs or chest CTAs performed since the date of the patient's last screening CT should also be noted.

6.2 Standardized Reporting Protocols and National Registry Requirements

The goal in LCS is to identify early curable lung cancer. Early lung cancer usually manifests as a small lung nodule. When reporting a nodule, the radiologist describes the size, character (solid, part-solid, or nonsolid), margins, and location of the nodule. If a prior CT is available, the radiologist determines if the nodule is new, growing, getting smaller, or remaining stable. Changes in the solid component of a part-solid are especially important to assess.

The Lung CT Screening Reporting & Data System (Lung-RADS) was adopted by the American College of Radiology in 2014 [6]. This structured reporting system allows for uniform reporting and consistency in exam interpretation. Recent evidence-based updates to Lung-RADS have also helped decrease the false positive rates.

The Lung-RADS assessment categories from 1 through 4 are based on the exam findings and features of any nodules identified [Fig. 6.1]. The categories

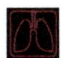

Lung-RADS® Version 1.1

Assessment Categories Release date: 2019

Category Descriptor	Lung-RADS Score	Findings	Management	Risk of Malignancy	Est. Population Prevalence
Incomplete	0	Prior chest CT examination(s) being located for comparison Part or all of lungs cannot be evaluated	Additional lung cancer screening CT images and/or comparison to prior chest CT examinations is needed	n/a	1%
Negative No nodules and definitely benign nodules	1	No lung nodules Nodule(s) with specific calcifications: complete, central, popcorn, concentric rings and fat containing nodules			
Benign Appearance or Behavior Nodules with a very low likelihood of becoming a clinically active cancer due to size or lack of growth	2	**Perifissural nodule(s)** *(See Footnote 11)* < 10 mm (524 mm³) **Solid nodule(s):** < 6 mm (< 113 mm³) new < 4 mm (< 34 mm³) **Part solid nodule(s):** < 6 mm total diameter (< 113 mm³) on baseline screening **Non solid nodule(s) (GGN):** <30 mm (<14137 mm³) **OR** ≥ 30 mm (≥ 14137 mm³) and unchanged or slowly growing **Category 3 or 4 nodules unchanged for ≥ 3 months**	Continue annual screening with LDCT in 12 months	< 1%	90%
Probably Benign Probably benign finding(s) - short term follow up suggested; includes nodules with a low likelihood of becoming a clinically active cancer	3	**Solid nodule(s):** ≥ 6 to < 8 mm (≥ 113 to < 268 mm³) at baseline **OR** new 4 mm to < 6 mm (34 to < 113 mm³) **Part solid nodule(s)** ≥ 6 mm total diameter (≥ 113 mm³) with solid component < 6 mm (< 113 mm³) **OR** new < 6 mm total diameter (< 113 mm³) **Non solid nodule(s)** (GGN) ≥ 30 mm (≥ 14137 mm³) on baseline CT or new	6 month LDCT	1-2%	5%
Suspicious Findings for which additional diagnostic testing is recommended	4A	**Solid nodule(s):** ≥ 8 to < 15 mm (≥ 268 to < 1767 mm³) at baseline **OR** growing < 8 mm (< 268 mm³) **OR** new 6 to < 8 mm (113 to < 268 mm³) **Part solid nodule(s):** ≥ 6 mm (≥ 113 mm³) with solid component ≥ 6 mm to < 8 mm (≥ 113 to < 268 mm³) **OR** with a new or growing < 4 mm (< 34 mm³) solid component **Endobronchial nodule**	3 month LDCT; PET/CT may be used when there is a ≥ 8 mm (≥ 268 mm³) solid component	5-15%	2%
Very Suspicious Findings for which additional diagnostic testing and/or tissue sampling is recommended	4B	**Solid nodule(s)** ≥ 15 mm (≥ 1767 mm³) **OR** new or growing, and ≥ 8 mm (≥ 268 mm³) **Part solid nodule(s) with:** a solid component ≥ 8 mm (≥ 268 mm³) **OR** a new or growing ≥ 4 mm (≥ 34 mm³) solid component	Chest CT with or without contrast, PET/CT and/or tissue sampling depending on the *probability of malignancy and comorbidities. PET/CT may be used when there is a ≥ 8 mm (≥ 268 mm³) solid component. For new large nodules that develop on an annual repeat screening CT, a 1 month LDCT may be recommended to address potentially infectious or inflammatory conditions	> 15%	2%
	4X	Category 3 or 4 nodules with additional features or imaging findings that increases the suspicion of malignancy			
Other Clinically Significant or Potentially Clinically Significant Findings (non lung cancer)	S	**Modifier - may add on to category 0-4 coding**	As appropriate to the specific finding	n/a	10%

IMPORTANT NOTES FOR USE:
1) Negative screen: does not mean that an individual does not have lung cancer
2) Size: To calculate nodule mean diameter, measure both the long and short axis to one decimal point, and report mean nodule diameter to one decimal point
3) Size Thresholds: apply to nodules at first detection, and that grow and reach a higher size category
4) Growth: an increase in size of > 1.5 mm (> 2 mm³)
5) Exam Category: each exam should be coded 0-4 based on the nodule(s) with the highest degree of suspicion
6) Exam Modifiers: S modifier may be added to the 0-4 category
7) Lung Cancer Diagnosis: Once a patient is diagnosed with lung cancer, further management (including additional imaging such as PET/CT) may be performed for purposes of lung cancer staging; this is no longer screening
8) Practice audit definitions: a negative screen is defined as categories 1 and 2; a positive screen is defined as categories 3 and 4
9) Category 4B Management: this is predicated on the probability of malignancy based on patient evaluation, patient preference and risk of malignancy; radiologists are encouraged to use the McWilliams et al assessment tool when making recommendations
10) Category 4X: nodules with additional imaging findings that increase the suspicion of lung cancer, such as spiculation, GGN that doubles in size in 1 year, enlarged lymph nodes etc
11) Solid nodules with smooth margins, an oval, lentiform or triangular shape, and maximum diameter less than 10 mm or 524 mm³ (perifissural nodules) should be classified as category 2
12) Category 3 and 4A nodules that are unchanged on interval CT should be coded as category 2, and individuals returned to screening in 12 months
13) LDCT: low dose chest CT

*Additional resources available at - https://www.acr.org/Clinical-Resources/Reporting-and-Data-Systems/Lung-Rads
*Link to Lung-RADS calculator - https://brocku.ca/lung-cancer-screening-and-risk-prediction/risk-calculators/

ACR®
RADIOLOGY
QUALITY IS OUR IMAGE

Fig. 6.1 Structured reporting system in Lung-RADS Version 1.1

range from negative or benign in appearance (Lung-RADS 1 and 2) to probably benign (Lung-RADS 3) to suspicious (Lung-RADS 4). The Lung-RADS system includes management recommendations based on the risk of malignancy. The majority of patients (approximately 80–90%) receive a Lung-RADS 1 or 2 and a recommendation to continue annual screening with a follow-up chest CT in 12 months. Patients receiving a Lung-RADS 3 or 4A receive a recommendation to return for a follow-up CT in 6 months or 3 months. The most suspicious nodules categorized as 4B or 4X need more immediate workup, typically either a PET-CT or tissue sampling.

The International Early Lung Cancer Action Program ELCAP (IELCAP) uses a slightly different reporting strategy [7]. The IELCAP protocol pre-dates Lung-RADS and has informed many of the decision points in lung cancer screening [Fig. 6.2]. Both Lung-RADS and IELCAP evaluate nodule consistency (solid, part-solid, and nonsolid) and use a 6 mm size threshold for solid nodules for a "positive" exam [6, 7]. Both strategies provide management recommendations, whether indicating the need for immediate workup or follow-up imaging.

Even if no suspicious lung nodules are identified, the presence of smoking-related lung disease including emphysema and bronchitis should be reported. Other smoking-related abnormalities such as coronary artery calcification and osteoporosis should be described. The presence of these findings can help encourage smoking cessation or maintenance of cessation. Enrollment in LCS and showing patients evidence of smoking-related tissue damage on their chest CTs are considered teachable moments for smoking cessation [8].

Medicare reimbursement originally required submission of data to a national registry but this is now optional. The only CMS approved registry is the ACR's Lung Cancer Screening Registry (LCSR) [9]. The LCSR is a quality assurance tool which monitors compliance with patient eligibility criteria, radiation dose, incidental findings, patient adherence to annual screening, and radiologist reporting patterns. It is the only available tool for gathering data at the national level and assessing quality metrics in LCS.

Tracking patient information, exam results, and follow-up data can be challenging. Initially, programs often use chart review and computer-based spreadsheets to gather and record this info. However, as programs grow and more patients are enrolled each year, more robust strategies are needed. Programs may use homegrown data management tools or commercial software. Regardless of the tool used, a tracking system is necessary to monitor and ensure patient care is timely and appropriate.

An additional reporting responsibility in LCS is sending a summary of the CT results directly to the patient. The CT results with a cover letter containing patient-oriented language should be sent to the patient and the ordering provider. In accordance with the International Association for the Study of Lung Cancer (IASLC) guidelines, the use of "person-first" language is recommended. This language puts the person before the disease and describes what the person has, not who the person is [10]. For example, instead of identifying a patient as a "smoker," the patient is described as a "person who smokes."

IELCAP Baseline Screening Protocol

Negative: No nodules, RETURN FOR ANNUAL REPEAT   IELCAP = 1

Semi-Positive: RETURN FOR ANNUAL REPEAT   IELCAP = 2

  a. Only nonsolid nodules, regardless of size, or
  b. Largest solid, part-solid (solid component) < 6.0 mm,
  c. Peri-fissural nodules< 10.0 mm in diameter with smooth margin and lentiform, oval, or triangular shape;
  d. Costal pleural nodules<10.0 mm in diameter with smooth margin and any shape (lenticular, oval, semi-circular, triangular, polygonal, or round shape); other than irregular.

Indeterminate: RETURN FOR LDCT IN 3 MONTHS   IELCAP = 3

  a. Largest solid, part-solid (solid component) 6.0-14.9 mm when follow-up CT scan in 3 months after baseline shows growth at a nonmalignant rate, RETURN 9 MONTHS LATER FOR FIRST ANNUAL REPEAT.

Positive: IELCAP = 4

  a. Largest solid, part-solid (solid component) 6.0-14.9 mm in size after a follow-up CT scan in 3 months shows growth at a malignant rate;
  b. Largest solid or part-solid nodule 15.0 mm or larger;
  c. Solid endobronchial nodule.

WORKUP OPTIONS FOR POSITIVE RESULTS:

A) If the nodule appearance is highly suggestive of lung cancer, immediate biopsy is recommended.
B) Another option is to perform PET scan, particularly if the solid component of the nodule is 10.0 or more mm in diameter. If the PET result is positive, biopsy is recommended, but if negative or indeterminate a low-dose CT 1-3 months later is performed. If there is growth, biopsy is recommended, but if there is partial or complete resolution on CT, the workup stops.
C) When multiple nodules are present and occult infection or inflammation is a possibility, an added option is a course of a broad spectrum antibiotic with anaerobic coverage followed by low-dose CT 1-3 months later (72). The result is acted on as specified in option B.
D) If an endobronchial nodule is identified at the time of the initial CT, the participant is asked to cough vigorously several times and the region of interest is reimaged at that time. If the endobronchial nodule is not recognized at the time of the baseline CT scan, the participant is recalled for a follow-up low-dose CT within one month. At the time of the follow-up CT scan, the participant is asked to cough vigorously several times. If the nodule is still present, the participant is referred for pulmonary consultation, and if necessary, bronchoscopy. If classic features of retained secretions are identified such as low attenuation, air bubbles, stranding and multiplicity, call back is not necessary [also see NCCN Guidelines 2016 (92)].

Fig. 6.2 Structured reporting system in IELCAP

6.3 Managing Screening Findings on Lung Cancer Screening CTs

Ideally screening should be performed within a multidisciplinary program with a team-based approach. Best practice LCS strategies utilize a multidisciplinary team including LCS program coordinators/patient navigators, CT technologists, radiologists, primary care providers, advanced practice providers (APPs), pulmonologists, thoracic surgeons, medical oncologists, radiation oncologists, and pathologists.

With the use of structured reporting as outlined in the previous section, the radiologist provides follow-up recommendations. Most commonly the recommendation is to continue annual screening with a follow-up low-dose chest CT in 12 months. Diagnostic CT follow-up in 3 or 6 months is typically recommended for the "positive CTs," the Lung-RADS 4A and Lung-RADS 3 cases. For the Lung-RADS 4B and Lung-RADS 4X cases, care is escalated with a recommendation for more immediate workup with a PET-CT or tissue sampling or occasionally a 1 month follow-up chest CT.

A Multidisciplinary Suspicious Lung Nodule Conference is valuable for the review of patients with suspicious nodules in the Lung-RADS 4 category. The Suspicious Lung Nodule Conference can be held immediately after the Lung Tumor Board since most of the key participants are already assembled. The referring provider should be invited to attend, either in-person or by calling in to a virtual meeting. Coordination of the Suspicious Lung Nodule Conference may be done by the LCS Program Coordinators or other LCS support staff. A process needs to be in place to compile the list of cases to be sent to the person presenting the Conference, usually the radiologist.

Within a centralized LCS Program, the program staff help manage the care continuum. They call results to the patients, answer questions and explain the rationale for any needed follow-up care. For patients needing escalation in care, either program staff or the referring provider, depending on the structure of the program, will discuss the findings with the patient. For the Lung-RADS 4 cases, the provider or program staff lets the patient know their case is going to be discussed at the upcoming Nodule Conference.

In settings where a Nodule Conference is not feasible, referral of the suspicious nodules to a Nodule Clinic or a local referral center is an alternative. A process needs to be in place so that the list of patients with suspicious nodules is communicated to the Clinic or facility in a timely fashion.

Whether cases are managed in a Nodule Conference, Nodule Clinic, or referral center, the expectation is that the providers have expertise and experience in lung nodule management. In addition, the providers may use risk prediction models to help determine the risk of malignancy in particular nodules. Based on the appearance of the nodule and clinical history, the tools usually involve risk calculators that estimate the likelihood that a nodule is malignant [11–13]. This additional information can enhance medical decision making and help guide the aggressiveness of recommended next steps. Importantly, communication about the recommendations from the Nodule Conference needs to occur so a plan for going forward is documented. The overarching goal is to provide the most appropriate timely care for the patient to optimize survival and quality of life.

Tracking the diagnostic follow-up exams on screening patients can be a challenge. Many LCS Programs find it useful to create a specific order and exam title for the follow-up LCS CTs. For example, the follow-up CT for a screen detected nodule might be called "CT Chest LCS Follow-up." The exam is a diagnostic chest CT with CPT code 71250 but has a more specific title than the usual "CT Chest WO." This allows the ordering and completion of the follow-up exams to be tracked. The "CT Chest LCS Follow-up" exams should be done with the same protocol as the low-dose screening CT to minimize radiation dose and to optimize comparison with the prior study. A Lung-RADS score should be added to the dictation so that the patient can continue to be tracked through the lung screening program.

6.4 Managing Incidental Findings on Lung Cancer Screening CT

In addition to identifying early stage lung cancer, LCS also provides an opportunity to identify significant and potentially significant incidental findings (IFs). Since LCS includes cross-sectional imaging of the entire chest, from the lower neck to the upper abdomen, multiple organs are visualized or partially visualized. There is an opportunity therefore to detect cardiovascular disease, aortic abnormalities, pulmonary disease including COPD and interstitial lung disease, as well as extrapulmonary neoplasms in the thyroid, mediastinum, esophagus, kidney, liver, pancreas, and breast. LCS CT can also identify fatty infiltration of the liver and low bone density, compatible with osteopenia or osteoporosis [14, 15].

IFs on LCS CT are common. Some IFs are significant and considered "actionable" while others are considered insignificant and require no follow-up. An "actionable" IF requires follow-up to determine if a lesion is benign or malignant (such as a renal mass) or if the patient may benefit from a clinical intervention (such as a statin drug for coronary artery calcium). The frequency of incidental findings varies substantially depending on how they are defined. Studies have reported a wide range of IFs, varying from 4 to 94% [16–19]. The variability relates to no consistent definition of what constitutes an IF and which IFs are considered actionable. The reported frequency of actionable IFs varies from 1 to 20% [20].

The most common IFs in LCS are pulmonary abnormalities and cardiovascular disease [19–23]. Morgan et al. reported the most common IFs are respiratory (69.6%), cardiovascular (67.5%), and GI (25.9%) [23]. In their review, nearly all patients had at least one IF reported but only 15% were actionable. Interestingly, although many patients had respiratory IFs, such as emphysema (50.6%) and bronchial wall thickening (39.4%), only 1.8% of the pulmonary findings led to additional evaluation. In contrast, 15.3% of cardiovascular IFs led to a referral to Cardiology.

The low number of follow-up evaluations for pulmonary findings is surprising as only 32% of the patients had known COPD. Although emphysema is not considered an "actionable finding," many patients might have benefited from a pulmonary referral since early intervention can improve outcomes for patients with COPD [24].

Cardiovascular disease was the leading cause of death in the NLST [21]. The presence of coronary artery calcification (CAC) correlates with the risk of subsequent cardiovascular events. The high number of patients with coronary artery calcification is expected as smoking is a known risk factor for cardiovascular disease. Although the most accurate assessment of CAC is done with ECG-gated CT, CAC can be effectively measured on non-gated LDCT [25].

The need for follow-up of solid organ lesions relates to the low-dose technique used in LCS which does not optimally demonstrate soft tissues and frequently only portions of an organ are visualized, particularly in the abdomen. The follow-up exam needs to completely image the organ of concern and may require intravenous contrast. Fortunately, the prevalence of extrapulmonary malignancies in LCS is low, with reports indicating 0–1.6% [21, 25–27]. Nguyen et al. reported 67 of 17,309 LCS patients (0.39%) had primary extrathoracic cancers diagnosed during screening [19]. Rampinelli et al. identified extrathoracic malignancies in 27 of 5201 participants in the COSMOS (Continuous Observation of Smoking Subjects) study [27]. The most commonly diagnosed cancers were renal, thyroid, and lymphoma [19, 27].

Follow-up rates for IFs in LCS are variable and guidelines are needed to better define potentially significant abnormalities [18]. There are no internationally agreed upon recommendations for handling IFs [28]. Ideally, the CT report should indicate which of the IFs are actionable. There is, unfortunately, inconsistency in radiologist reporting and the reports may lack clear concise recommendations for follow-up [18]. The variability in definition and radiologist reporting of incidental findings can lead to confusion on the part of the LCS program coordinators who often help manage the care continuum for the LCS patients. Moreover, the responsibility for following up on incidental findings often falls to the patient's PCP who may be uncertain about whether an abnormality described in the report requires referral or further imaging.

The American College of Radiology has developed several White Papers to assist with interpretation of findings on CT [29–34]. The complexity and lack of immediate accessibility of these documents may present a barrier to their routine use, especially among LCS navigators and PCPs. To address this concern, the ACR's Lung Cancer Screening Steering Committee developed a Quick Guide on managing IFs in LCS (Fig. 6.3). The guide was developed with subspecialty expert review and is based on published evidence or consensus documents. The goal was to provide quick and easy access to IF management recommendations for LCS program navigators and primary care providers. The document outlines common IFs, describes the significance of such abnormalities and provides recommended workup or next steps when needed.

Detection of IFs may reduce morbidity and mortality in some LCS patients but unnecessary testing and treatment may also occur [26, 35, 36]. Screening programs should develop a standard approach for evaluation of the IFs. Using tools such as the

ACR® Lung Cancer Screening CT Incidental Findings
Quick Reference Guide

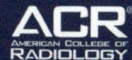

This Quick Guide is intended for use by Lung Cancer Screening (LCS) program coordinators and nurse navigators as they assist in the care coordination of LCS patients in collaboration with the referring providers.

- The Quick Guide lists common incidental findings on LCS CT and the typical management and/or appropriate follow–up recommendations.
- Comparison to prior exams is important to assess for stability or change.
- The guidance provided is intended to serve as a simple reference tool and does not replace the more comprehensive White Paper, ACR Appropriateness Criteria® and reference documents listed on the third page.
- The interpreting radiologist should include significant incidental findings that need attention, with recommended follow-up, in the "Impression" section of the report.
- Questions about the findings in a radiology report are best answered by the radiologist who interpreted the exam.

Legend/Abbreviations:

ASCVD = atherosclerotic cardiovascular disease
CAC = coronary artery calcification
CE = contrast enhanced
CT = computed tomography
→ = action recommended, text in **Bold** type

MR = magnetic resonance imaging
OK = typically, but not always, insignificant or benign
US = ultrasound
w/u: = work up with follow-up imaging
PCP = primary care provider

Anatomic Region	Findings/Recommendations
Abdominal	
Adrenal[1]	• Adrenal calcification – OK. • Nodule < 10 HU (fat density), likely adenoma – OK. • Soft tissue density nodule < 1 cm – OK. • Adrenal nodule stable ≥ 1 year – OK. → **Any other nodule or mass → w/u: CE Adrenal CT or MRI.**
Kidney[2]	• Non-obstructing renal calculi – OK. • Simple or hyperdense/hemorrhagic cyst ("Bosniak 1 or 2") < 4 cm – OK. → **Soft tissue density (or mixed density) renal mass → w/u: CT or MRI of the Kidneys without and with IV contrast.**
Liver[3]	• Simple cyst – OK. • Nodule < 1 cm – OK, likely benign. → **Soft tissue nodule/mass ≥ 1cm → w/u: CE Abdomen CT or MRI.** → **Fatty liver/hepatic steatosis or cirrhosis → PCP evaluation.**
Pancreas[4]	• Coarse calcifications – OK. → **Cyst/mass → w/u: CE Abdomen CT or MRI.**
Musculoskeletal	
Bone Density[13,14,15]	• > 130 HU at L1 – OK. → **100 – 130 HU at L1 (Osteopenia) → consider PCP evaluation.** → **< 100 HU at L1 (Osteoporosis) → PCP evaluation and consider DEXA.**
Other	• Degenerative disc disease – OK.

Fig. 6.3 The ACR Lung Cancer Screening CT Incidental Findings Quick Reference Guide

Cardiovascular	
Aorta[6]	• "Ectasia of the thoracic aorta" – OK. • Mural calcification – OK. • Ascending Aorta < 42mm – OK. → **Ascending Aorta ≥ 42 mm → PCP surveillance or cardiology consult for aneurysm surveillance.**
Cardiac/pericardium	• Trace/small pericardial effusion – OK. → **Moderate or large pericardial effusion → discuss with PCP.** → **Other Abnormalities (such as moderate or greater aortic valve calcification) → PCP evaluation.**
Coronary arteries[7,8]	• Coronary artery calcifications (CAC) typically reported as none, mild, moderate, or severe. → **CAC present → PCP evaluation for ASCVD risk assessment.**
Main PA measurement[9,10]	• < 31 mm – OK. • → **31 mm → PCP evaluation, consider Cardiology or Pulmonary consult.**
Breast	
	• Coarse calcifications – OK. • Cyst with no associated solid component – OK. → **Any other nodule/mass or asymmetric density → w/u: diagnostic mammogram +/- US.**
Esophagus	
	→ **Large hiatal hernia or dilated esophagus → PCP evaluation.** → **Focal wall thickening or mass → PCP evaluation, consider GI consult.**
Lung/Pleura	
Lung[11]	• Atelectasis – mild/subsegmental – OK. • Emphysema/bronchial wall thickening (Expected findings) – consider PCP evaluation; may benefit from Pulmonary consult. → **Fibrotic interstitial lung disease (ILD) → recommend pulmonary consultation.** → **Bronchiectasis/ground glass opacity/cystic lung disease/diffuse nodular disease → PCP evaluation, consider pulmonary consultation.**
Pleura	→ **New disease – effusion, thickening, mass → PCP evaluation, consider pulmonary consultation.**
Mediastinum	
Lymph nodes (Short axis measurement)[12]	• < 15 mm – OK. → **≥ 15 mm & no explainable cause → PCP evaluation; consider pulmonary consultation. Consider follow-up CE Chest CT in 3–6 months.**
Other[12]	• Cyst – OK. → **Mass (soft tissue or mixed density) → CE Chest MRI or CT.**
Thyroid[16]	
Features	• Large and heterogeneous, likely goiter – probably OK; consider thyroid function testing. • Nodule < 15 mm – OK. → **Nodule ≥ 15 mm or with suspicious features → w/u: thyroid US and clinical evaluation.**

Link to the ACR white papers on incidental findings:
https://publish.smartsheet.com/42d18e874a164318a0f702481f2fbb70

Fig. 6.3 (continued)

References:

1) Mayo-Smith WW, Song JH, Boland GL, et al. Management of Incidental Adrenal Masses: ACR Incidental Findings Committee. *J Am Coll Radiol*. 2017 Aug;14(8):1038–1044.
2) Herts BR, Silverman SG, Hindman NM, et al. Management of the Incidental Renal Mass on CT: ACR Incidental Findings Committee. *J Am Coll Radiol*. 2018 Feb;15(2):264–273.
3) Gore RM, Pickhardt PJ, Mortele KJ, et al. Management of Incidental Liver Lesions on CT: ACR Incidental Findings Committee. *J Am Coll Radiol*. 2017 Nov;14(11):1429–1437.
4) Megibow AJ, Baker ME, Morgan DE, et al. Management of Incidental Pancreatic Cysts: ACR Incidental Findings Committee. *J Am Coll Radiol*. 2017 Jul;14(7):911–923.
5) Heller MT, Harisinghani M, Neitlich JD, Yeghiayan P, Berland LL. Managing Incidental Findings on Abdominal and Pelvic CT and MRI, Part 3: White Paper of the ACR Incidental Findings Committee II on Splenic and Nodal Findings. *J Am Coll Radiol*. 2013 Nov;10(11):833–839.
6) McComb BL, Munden RF, Duan F, Jain AA, Tuite C, Chiles C. Normative reference values of thoracic aortic diameter in American College of Radiology Imaging Network (ACRIN 6654) arm of National Lung Cancer Screening Trial. *Clin Imaging*. 2016;40(5):936–943.
7) Hecht HS, Cronin P, Blaha MJ, et al. 2016 SCCT/STR Guidelines for Coronary Artery Calcium Scoring Of Noncontrast Noncardiac Chest CT Scans: A Report Of The Society Of Cardiovascular Computed Tomography And Society Of Thoracic Radiology. *J Cardiovasc Comput Tomogr*. 2017:11(1):74–84.
8) Arnett DK, Blumenthal RS, Albert MA, et al. 2019 ACC/AHA Guideline on the Primary Prevention of Cardiovascular Disease: A Report of the American College of Cardiology/American Heart Association Task Force on Clinical Practice Guidelines. *Circulation* 2019 Sep;140(11):e596–e646.
9) Truong QA, Bhatia HS, Szymonifka J, et al. A four-tier classification system of pulmonary artery metrics on computed tomography for the diagnosis and prognosis of pulmonary hypertension. *J Cardiovasc Comput Tomogr*. 2018;12(1):60–66.
10) Truong QA, Massaro JM, Rogers IS, et al. Reference values for normal pulmonary artery dimensions by noncontrast cardiac computed tomography: the Framingham Heart Study. *Circ Cardiovasc Imaging*. 2012 Jan;5(1):147–154.
11) Munden RF, Black WC, Hartman TE, et al. Managing Incidental Findings on Thoracic CT: Lung Findings. A White Paper of the ACR Incidental Findings Committee. *J Am Coll Radiol*. 2021 Jul;S1546-1440(21)00376–8.
12) Munden RF, Carter BW, Chiles C, et al. Managing Incidental Findings on Thoracic CT: Mediastinal and Cardiovascular Findings. A White Paper of the ACR Incidental Findings Committee. *J Am Coll Radiol*. 2018 Aug;15(8):1087–1096.
13) Lee SJ, Pickhardt PJ. Opportunistic Screening for Osteoporosis Using Body CT Scans Obtained for Other Indications: the UW Experience. *Clinic Rev Bone Miner Metab*. 2017; 15(3):128–137.
14) Buckens CF, van der Graaf Y, Verkooijen HM, et al. Osteoporosis Markers on Low-Dose Lung Cancer Screening Chest Computed Tomography Scans Predict All-Cause Mortality. *Eur Radiol*. 2015 Jan;25(1):132–139.
15) Boutin RD, Lenchik L. Value-Added Opportunistic CT: Insights into Osteoporosis and Sarcopenia. *AJR*. 2020;215:582–594.
16) Hoang JK, Langer JE, Middleton WD, et al. Managing Incidental Thyroid Nodules Detected on Imaging: White Paper of The ACR Incidental Thyroid Findings Committee. *J Am Coll Radiol*. 2015 Feb;12(2):143–150.

Fig. 6.3 (continued)

Quick Reference Guide helps ensure patients receive appropriate follow-up and helps minimize unnecessary diagnostic workup. The potential benefits and harms resulting from the investigation of IFs should also be part of the SDM discussion [37].

Appropriate reporting and management of IFs on LCS CT have the potential to improve health outcomes and cost-effectiveness in LCS.

6.5   Updates in Lung Cancer Screening Technology

Rapidly occurring advances in technology have the potential to increase the efficiency of lung cancer screening, improve the early detection and optimize treatment of lung cancer.

Computer-aided detection (CAD) tools for CT have been available for several years. CAD can aid in the diagnosis of lung nodules, detecting some that are missed by the radiologist. These tools typically allow for rapid identification of nodules but were not enthusiastically adopted due to a high number of false positives. In addition, the review of nodule candidates often was time consuming and prolonged image interpretation.

Volumetric measurements of nodules through CAD are useful and can help guide management. Volume measurements and Volume Doubling Times (VDTs) have been shown to more accurately assess nodule growth and guide follow-up [38, 39]. For example, diagnostic workup is typically recommended rather than follow-up CT for a VDT of <400 days.

Artificial Intelligence (AI) is a broad term that typically refers to computer systems that can interpret and learn from data to perform certain tasks and reach certain goals [40]. AI tools including the use of machine learning, deep learning, and convolutional neural networks allow for the automatic characterization and classification of lung nodules [41]. Tools for AI can be presented to the radiologist as a first, concurrent or second read. AI can also be used to evaluate coronary artery calcium (CAC) with high sensitivity and specificity [42].

Radiomics is a rapidly evolving field that extracts features from medical images and translates them into manageable data for predictive analytics [43]. Radiomics not only analyzes common nodule features of size, shape, and CT density but also evaluates texture, wavelets, and entropy that cannot be evaluated with the human eye. Coupled with AI, radiomics can handle massive amounts of data. Combined with genomics, plasma biomarkers, and histologic patterns, radiomics has been shown to help differentiate between benign and malignant nodules [44].

Several biomarkers have been investigated that may be able to improve early detection or identify high risk individuals. These include exhaled breath, autoantibodies, complement fragments, cell-free nucleic acids, DNA methylation, and blood protein profiles. Some studies have suggested that biomarkers may be able to personalize screening intervals such as occurring every other year as opposed to annual screening [45]. It is generally agreed biomarkers for LCS need further investigation.

AI, radiomics and biomarkers offer a promising approach which may increase sensitivity, specificity, and accuracy in LCS.

6.6   Women and Lung Cancer Screening

Lung cancer kills more women annually than breast, ovarian, and cervical cancer combined [46]. Over the last 42 years, the incidence of lung cancer decreased by 36% in men while increasing 84% in women [47]. Despite these statistics, a nationwide survey in 2020 discovered that only 8% of adults know that lung cancer is the leading cancer killer of women [48]. Randomized-controlled trials have demonstrated a significant mortality benefit with annual low-dose CT (LDCT) for lung cancer screening, and several, including the National Lung Screening Trial (NLST) and the Dutch NELSON trial, have shown disproportionately higher benefit among women [21, 39]. The more recently published German Lung Cancer Screening Intervention (LUSI) study reported a 69% reduction in mortality in lung cancer in women compared to 6% in men [49].

The study and implementation of lung cancer screening has unfortunately not yet adequately raised awareness of lung cancer in the female population. Women have been historically underrepresented in clinical trials [50] which remained true in lung cancer screening trials. This included the NLST which enrolled 41% female participants and the NELSON trial which enrolled only 16% [39, 51]. Clinical implementation of lung screening has also been more challenging for women. While efforts to improve lung screening rates nationwide are underway [52, 53], women are significantly less likely than men to be offered lung screening by healthcare providers [54].

Disparities exist not only in who is offered screening, but also in populations meeting screening eligibility criteria. Numerous studies evaluating the clinical implementation of lung cancer screening have demonstrated a significant disparity in patient screening eligibility, particularly in women and underrepresented minorities [55–57]. This in part led to the new guideline recommendations for the expansion of lung screening to younger individuals with less tobacco exposure published in 2021 [1]. The Cancer Intervention and Surveillance Modeling Network (CISNET) Lung Cancer Screening Working Group has estimated that this guideline expansion will increase the relative proportion of women in the screening eligible population by 96% [58].

Lung cancer appears to be a different disease in women, with several studies demonstrating variation in the histological distribution of lung tumors between sexes [59–61]. For example, among women with lung cancer, the incidence rate of lung cancer in nonsmoking women is between 14.4% and 20.8%, compared to 4.8%–13.7% in nonsmoking men [62]. In addition to being more susceptible to lung cancer as non-smokers, women have also been shown to be more susceptible than men to the carcinogenic effects of cigarettes [63]. Lung cancer is now more common among young women than men; the increased incidence in women cannot be explained by differences in smoking behavior alone [64].

Women therefore present a population where lung cancer screening may be enormously effective as they are seeing increased rates of lung cancer as compared to men and have been shown to have a greater mortality benefit when screened for lung cancer. Currently, participation in lung cancer screening by both men and women is discouragingly low, with less than 15% of eligible individuals estimated to have enrolled in a lung screening program nationwide [65]. Targeted intervention strategies are needed to improve enrollment in lung screening programs especially for women who are less likely than men to be offered lung screening. One such strategy is capitalizing on the success of screening mammography to improve awareness of screening for lung cancer. The CDC has reported up to 70% of women over age 40 have had a mammogram in the past 2 years [66]. Mammography thus offers a "teachable moment" for women to be informed both of their eligibility for lung screening and its benefits. Research has demonstrated that roughly 7% of women engaged in breast screening are lung screening eligible [67], and that among these women, a significant number are in fact dying from lung cancer [68].

The two big questions for women and lung screening remain (1) what the ideal eligible screening population is and (2) how to engage and enroll those who are eligible in lung screening programs. The expansion of the lung screening eligibility criteria by the USPSTF in 2021 was a critical step in reducing disparities in screening eligibility for women. The question remains whether this is enough, as young women with even less tobacco exposure continue to be diagnosed with and die from lung cancer. There is particular interest in evaluating lung cancer in women, as the incidence of lung cancer in women without a significant smoking history is greater than in men [62, 69]. As of yet, screening is not recommended for anyone younger than age 50 and with less than a 20 pack-year history, though several trials conducted in Asia have shown success in screening for lung cancer in women without a history of tobacco use [70–72].

While guidelines will continue to be studied and revised, it is critical that women who are eligible for lung screening are made aware of the availability of this life-saving exam. The fact remains that lung cancer is the leading cause of cancer-related mortality in women, and that screening women for lung cancer can save their lives.

References

1. US Preventive Services Task Force. Screening for lung cancer US Preventive Services Task Force Recommendation Statement. JAMA. 2021;325:962–70.
2. Centers for Medicare & Medicaid Services. Decision memo for screening for lung cancer with low dose computed tomography (LDCT) (CAG-00439N). 2015. https://www.cms.gov/medicare-coverage-database/details/nca-decision-memo.
3. Tammimagi MC, Katki HA, Hocking WG, et al. Selection criteria for lung-cancer screening. N Engl J Med. 2013;368:728–36.
4. Tammimagi MC, ten Haaf K, Toumazis I, et al. Development and validation of a multivariable Lung Cancer Risk Prediction Model that includes low-dose computed tomography screening results. JAMA Netw Open. 2019;2(3):e190204. https://doi.org/10.1001/jamanetworkopen.2019.0204.
5. Pasquinelli MM, Tammemagi MC, Kovitz KL, et al. Risk prediction model versus United States Preventive Services Task Force lung cancer screening eligibility criteria: reducing race disparities. J Thorac Oncol. 2020;15(11):1738–47.

6. American College of Radiology. Lung CT Screening Reporting & Data System (LungRADS Version 1.1). https://www.acr.org/LungRADS.
7. IELCAP. International v Early Lung Cancer Action Program: Screening Protocol. https://www.ielcap.org/Management.
8. Deppen SA, Grogan EL, Aldrich MC, Massion PP. Lung cancer screening and smoking cessation: a teachable moment. JNCI. 2014;106:1–2.
9. American College of Radiology. Lung Cancer Screening Registry. https://www.acr.org/LCSR.
10. IASLC Language Guide. 2021. IASLC. https://www.iaslc.orf/IASLCLanguageGuide.
11. McWillaims A, Tammemagi MC, Mayo JR, et al. Probability of lung cancer in pulmonary nodules detected on first screening CT. N Engl J Med. 2013;369:910–9.
12. White CS, Dharaiya E, Dalal S, et al. Vancouver risk calculator compared with ACR LungRADS in predicting malignancy: analysis of the National Lung Cancer Screening Trial. Radiology. 2019;291:205–11.
13. Choi HK, Ghobrial M, Mazzone PJ, et al. Models to estimate the probability of malignancy in patients with pulmonary nodules. Ann Am Thorac Soc. 2018;15(10):1117–26.
14. Penna R, Lim J, Williams BL, et al. Opportunistic screening of patients for hepatic steatosis: clinical follow-up and diagnostic yield. J Am Coll Radiol. 2021;18:1423–9.
15. Boutin RD, Lenchik L. Value-added opportunistic CT: insights into osteoporosis and sarcopenia. AJR. 2020;215:582–94.
16. Kinsinger LS, Anderson C, Kim J, et al. Implementation of lung cancer screening in the Veterans Health Administration. JAMA Intern Med. 2017;177(3):399–406.
17. Janssen K, Schertz K, Rubin N, Begnaud A. Incidental findings in a Decentralized Lung Cancer Screening Program. Ann Am Thorac Soc. 2019;16(9):1198–200.
18. Reiter MJ, Nemesure A, Madu E, et al. Frequency and distribution of incidental findings deemed appropriate for S modifier designation on low-dose CT in lung cancer screening program. Lung Cancer. 2018;120:1–6.
19. Nguyen XV, Davies L, Eastwood JD, Hoang JK. Extrapulmonary findings and malignancies in participants screened with chest CT in the National Lung Screening Trial. J Am Coll Radiol. 2017;14:324–30.
20. Tsai EB, Chiles C, Carter BW, et al. Incidental findings on lung cancer screening: significance and management. Semin Ultrasound CT MR. 2018;39:273–81.
21. The National Lung Screening Trial Research Team. Reduced lung-cancer mortality with low-dose computed tomographic screening. N Engl J Med. 2011;365:395–409.
22. Chung JH, Richards JC, Koelsch TL, et al. Screening for lung cancer: incidental pulmonary parenchymal findings. AJR. 2018;210:1–11.
23. Morgan L, Choi H, Reid M, Khawaja A, Mazzone PJ. Frequency of incidental findings and subsequent evaluation in low-dose computed tomographic scans for lung cancer screening. Ann Am Thorac Soc. 2017;14:1450–6.
24. Steiger D, Siddiqi MF, Yip R, et al. The importance of low-dose CT screening to identify emphysema in asymptomatic participants with and without a prior diagnosis of COPD. Clin Imaging. 2021;78:136–41.
25. Chiles C, Duan F, Gladish GW, et al. Association of coronary artery calcification and mortality in the national lung screening trial: a comparison of three scoring methods. Radiology. 2015;276(1):82–90.
26. Kucharczyk MJ, Menezes RJ, McGregor A, et al. Assessing the impact of incidental findings in a lung cancer screening study by using low-dose computed tomography. Can Assoc Radiol J. 2011;62:141–5.
27. Rampinelli C, Preda L, Maniglio M, et al. Extrapulmonary malignancies detected at lung cancer screening. Radiology. 2011;261:293–9.
28. Kauczor HU, Baird AM, Blum TG, et al. ESR/ERS statement paper on lung cancer screening. Eur Respir J. 2020;55(2):1900506. https://doi.org/10.1183/13993003.00506-2019.

29. Munden RF, Carter BW, Chiles C, et al. Managing incidental findings on thoracic CT: mediastinal and cardiovascular findings. A White Paper of the ACR Incidental Findings Committee. J Am Coll Radiol. 2018;15:1087–96.
30. Munden RF, Black WC, Hartman TE, et al. Managing incidental findings on thoracic CT: lung findings. A White Paper of the ACR Incidental Findings Committee. J Am Coll Radiol. 2021;18(9):1267–79.
31. Gore RM, Pickhardt PJ, Mortele KJ, et al. Management of incidental liver lesions on CT: a White paper of the ACR Incidental Findings Committee. Am Coll Radiol. 2017;13:1429–37.
32. Mayo-Smith WW, Song JH, Boland GL, et al. Management of incidental adrenal masses: a White Paper of the ACR Incidental Findings Committee. Am Coll Radiol. 2017;14:1038–44.
33. Herts BR, Silverman SG, Hindman NM, et al. Management of the incidental renal mass on CT: a White Paper of the ACR Incidental Findings Committee. Am Coll Radiol. 2018;15:264–73.
34. Megibow AJ, Baker ME, Morgan DE, et al. Management of the incidental pancreatic cysts: a White Paper of the ACR Incidental Findings Committee. Am Coll Radiol. 2017;14:911–23.
35. Gareen IF, Black WC, Tosteson TD, et al. Medical care cost were similar across the low-dose computed tomography and chest x-ray arms of the National Lung Screening Trial despite different rates of significant incidental findings. Med Care. 2018;56(5):403–9.
36. Gierada DS, Black WC, Chiles C, et al. Low-dose screening for lung cancer: evidence from 2 decades of study. Radiol Imaging Cancer. 2020;2(2):e190058. https://doi.org/10.1148/rycan.2020190058.
37. Godoy MCB, White CS, Erasmus JJ, et al. Extrapulmonary neoplasms in lung cancer screening. Transl Lung Cancer Res. 2018;7(3):368–75.
38. Horeweg N, van der Aalst CM, Vliegenthart R. Volumetric computed tomography for lung cancer: three rounds of the NELSON trial. Eur Respir J. 2013;42:1659–67.
39. De Koning HJ, van der Aalst CM, de Jong PA, et al. Reduced lung-cancer mortality with volume CT screening in a randomized trial. N Engl J Med. 2020;382:503–13.
40. Schreuder A, Scholten ET, van Ginneken B, Jacobs C. Artificial intelligence for detection and characterization of pulmonary nodules in lung cancer CT screening: ready for practice? Transl Lung Cancer Res. 2021;10(5):2378–88.
41. Mathew CJ, David AM, Mathew CMJ. Artificial intelligence and its future potential in lung cancer screening. EXCLI J. 2020;19:1552–62.
42. Chamberlin J, Kocher MR, Waltz J. Automated detection of lung nodules and coronary artery calcium using artificial intelligence on low-dose CT scans for lung cancer screening: accuracy and prognostic value. BMC Med. 2021;19(1):55. https://doi.org/10.1186/s12916-021-01928-3.
43. Binczyk F, Prazuch W, Bozek P, Polanska J. Radiomics and artificial intelligence in lung cancer screening. Transl Lung Cancer Rev. 2021;10(2):1186–99.
44. Espinoza JL, Dong LT. Artificial intelligence tools for refining lung cancer screening. J Clin Med. 2020;9:1–17.
45. Lam S, Tammemagi M. Contemporary issues in the implementation of lung cancer screening. Eur Respir Rev. 2021;30:1–17.
46. Siegel RL, Miller KD, Jemal A. Cancer statistics, 2018. CA Cancer J Clin. 2018;68(1):7–30. https://doi.org/10.3322/caac.21442. (In Eng)
47. Noone AM, Howlader N, Krapcho M, Miller D, Brest A, Yu M, Ruhl J, Tatalovich Z, Mariotto A, Lewis DR, Chen HS, Feuer EJ, Cronin KA, editors. SEER Cancer Statistics Review, 1975-2015. Bethesda, MD: National Cancer Institute. https://seer.cancer.gov/csr/1975_2015/, based on November 2017 SEER data submission, posted to the SEER web site, April 2018.
48. National Lung Health Barometer. LUNG FORCE. https://www.lung.org/lung-force/lung-health-barometer2020.
49. Becker N, Motsch E, Trotter A, et al. Lung cancer mortality reduction by LDCT screening-results from the randomized German LUSI trial. Int J Cancer. 2020;146(6):1503–13. https://doi.org/10.1002/ijc.32486. (In Eng)
50. Schiebinger L. Women's health and clinical trials. J Clin Invest. 2003;112(7):973–7. https://doi.org/10.1172/JCI19993. (In Eng)

51. National Lung Screening Trial Research T, Aberle DR, Adams AM, et al. Baseline characteristics of participants in the randomized national lung screening trial. J Natl Cancer Inst. 2010;102(23):1771–9. https://doi.org/10.1093/jnci/djq434. (In Eng)
52. Yong PC, Sigel K, Rehmani S, Wisnivesky J, Kale MS. Lung cancer screening uptake in the United States. Chest. 2020;157(1):236–8. https://doi.org/10.1016/j.chest.2019.08.2176.
53. Okereke IC, Nishi S, Zhou J, Goodwin JS. Trends in lung cancer screening in the United States, 2016-2017. J Thorac Dis. 2019;11(3):873–81. https://doi.org/10.21037/jtd.2019.01.105. (In Eng)
54. Warner ET, Lathan CS. Race and sex differences in patient provider communication and awareness of lung cancer screening in the health information National Trends Survey, 2013–2017. Prev Med. 2019;124:84–90. https://doi.org/10.1016/j.ypmed.2019.05.001.
55. Aldrich MC, Mercaldo SF, Sandler KL, Blot WJ, Grogan EL, Blume JD. Evaluation of USPSTF lung cancer screening guidelines among African American adult smokers. JAMA Oncol. 2019;5(9):1318–24. https://doi.org/10.1001/jamaoncol.2019.1402.
56. Ritzwoller DP, Meza R, Carroll NM, et al. Evaluation of population-level changes associated with the 2021 US force lung cancer screening recommendations in community-based health care systems. JAMA Netw Open. 2021;4(10):e2128176. https://doi.org/10.1001/jamanetworkopen.2021.28176.
57. Wu GX, Goldstein L, Kim JY, Raz DJ. Proportion of non-small-cell lung cancer patients that would have been eligible for lung cancer screening. Clin Lung Cancer. 2016;17(5):e131–9. https://doi.org/10.1016/j.cllc.2016.01.001. (In Eng)
58. Meza R, et al. Evaluation of the benefits and harms of lung cancer screening with low-dose computed tomography: a collaborative modeling study for the U.S. Preventive Services Task Force. (CISNET) and L. C. Work Group. Rockville, MD 20857. Agency for Healthcare Research and Quality. AHRQ Publication No. 20-05266-EF-2 July 2020: 177; 2020.
59. Patel JD, Bach PB, Kris MG. Lung cancer in US women: a contemporary epidemic. JAMA. 2004;291(14):1763–8. https://doi.org/10.1001/jama.291.14.1763.
60. Osann KE, Anton-Culver H, Kurosaki T, Taylor T. Sex differences in lung-cancer risk associated with cigarette smoking. Int J Cancer. 1993;54(1):44–8. https://doi.org/10.1002/ijc.2910540108.
61. Belani CP, Marts S, Schiller J, Socinski MA. Women and lung cancer: epidemiology, tumor biology, and emerging trends in clinical research. Lung Cancer. 2007;55(1):15–23. https://doi.org/10.1016/j.lungcan.2006.09.008.
62. Wakelee HA, Chang ET, Gomez SL, et al. Lung cancer incidence in never smokers. J Clin Oncol. 2007;25(5):472–8. https://doi.org/10.1200/JCO.2006.07.2983. (In Eng)
63. Shriver SP, Bourdeau HA, Gubish CT, et al. Sex-specific expression of gastrin-releasing peptide receptor: relationship to smoking history and risk of lung cancer. J Natl Cancer Inst. 2000;92(1):24–33. https://doi.org/10.1093/jnci/92.1.24. (In Eng)
64. Jemal A, Miller KD, Ma J, et al. Higher lung cancer incidence in young women than young men in the United States. N Engl J Med. 2018;378(21):1999–2009. https://doi.org/10.1056/NEJMoa1715907.
65. Maki KG, Shete S, Volk RJ. Examining lung cancer screening utilization with public-use data: opportunities and challenges. Prev Med. 2021;147:106503. https://doi.org/10.1016/j.ypmed.2021.106503. (In Eng)
66. Swan J, Breen N, Coates RJ, Rimer BK, Lee NC. Progress in cancer screening practices in the United States: results from the 2000 National Health Interview Survey. Cancer. 2003;97(6):1528–40. https://doi.org/10.1002/cncr.11208. (In Eng)
67. López DB, Flores EJ, Miles RC, et al. Assessing eligibility for lung cancer screening among women undergoing screening mammography: cross-sectional survey results from the National Health Interview Survey. J Am Coll Radiol. 2019;16(10):1433–9. https://doi.org/10.1016/j.jacr.2019.04.006.

68. Sandler KL, Haddad DN, Paulson AB, et al. Women screened for breast cancer are dying from lung cancer: an opportunity to improve lung cancer screening in a mammography population. J Med Screen. 2021;28(4):488–93. https://doi.org/10.1177/09691413211013058.
69. Lin KF, Wu HF, Huang WC, Tang PL, Wu MT, Wu FZ. Propensity score analysis of lung cancer risk in a population with high prevalence of non-smoking related lung cancer. BMC Pulm Med. 2017;17(1):120. https://doi.org/10.1186/s12890-017-0465-8. (In Eng)
70. Kim HY, Jung KW, Lim KY, et al. Lung cancer Screening with low-dose CT in female never smokers: retrospective cohort study with long-term national data follow-up. Cancer Res Treat. 2018;50(3):748–56. https://doi.org/10.4143/crt.2017.312. (In Eng)
71. Chien LH, Chen CH, Chen TY, et al. Predicting lung cancer occurrence in never-smoking females in Asia: TNSF-SQ, a prediction model. Cancer Epidemiol Biomark Prev. 2020;29(2):452–9. https://doi.org/10.1158/1055-9965.Epi-19-1221. (In Eng)
72. Kang HR, Cho JY, Lee SH, et al. Role of low-dose computerized tomography in lung cancer screening among never-smokers. J Thorac Oncol. 2019;14(3):436–44. https://doi.org/10.1016/j.jtho.2018.11.002. (In Eng)

Index